Praise for
Just Keep Breathing

An extraordinary journey told in a spiritually insightful way that will grip your heart and your emotions and cause you to take a step back and be grateful—that in some way, you will know Joan and indeed, yourself, a little better.

> Patti Machin Garrett,
> City Commissioner,
> Decatur, Georgia

There are many types and examples of bravery. In this true story by first-time author and educator Joan Curtis, you will experience how she coped on a daily basis with the challenge of her husband's battle with AIDs, the needs of their five children, and her own spiritual highs and lows of a life turned upside down. The honesty with which Curtis writes is sometimes painful and always surprising. It is a story that kept me turning pages because of this honesty. Above all, it is a triumphant love story that illustrates how one woman lived out the wedding promise of "til death do us part" and today continues to honor this love through the life she is living and the courage she is sharing. Her lesson is a simple one: If I can, you, also, can.

Carol Coulter,
Retired Educator

Joan Curtis has written courageously about courageous decisions. In the face of incredible pain, she faces each decision with honesty and strength—graciously accepting help when she needs it and generously sharing her strength when she sees others in need. From those daily decisions and conversations, she builds a network of love and support for everyone around her, and, when she needs it, that network supports her as well.

> Leslie Patterson, Ph. D.,
> Professor, University of North Texas
> College of Education

Despite the personal pain that Curtis had to endure, her words flow gently on the page as she shares her story of courage, tenacity, and caring.

> Carol D. Wickstrom, Ph. D.,
> Associate Professor, University of
> North Texas College of Education

With unflinching detail, Joan Curtis recounts the end of her husband's life and the ensuing devastation to her family. With humor, determination, and unconditional love for her children, Curtis demonstrates the power of hope and the strength of the human spirit.

> Julie Tolle, English Teacher,
> Billy Ryan High School

Just Keep Breathing

At 44, he died.
She didn't.

Joan Scott Curtis

Hugo House Publishers, Ltd.

Just Keep Breathing: At 44, he died. She didn't.
by Joan Scott Curtis

© 2013 Joan Scott Curtis

Published by:
Hugo House Publishers, Ltd.
Englewood, Colorado
Austin, Texas
877-700-0616
www.HugoHousePublishers.com

Book Design: Nick Zelinger, NZ Graphics

ISBN: 978-1-936449-56-9
Library of Congress Control Number: 2013930817

First Edition

Printed in the United States of America

For my grandchildren
Samantha, Alyssa, Dylan, Jordan, Austin,
Kiera, and Colby

This is the story of your Mimi.

Contents

Prologue

It was April 10th, Good Friday of 2009. I had flown to Lubbock, Texas, to witness the confirmation of my youngest son, Drew, into the Roman Catholic Church the evening before Easter. Drew had been reared in the Presbyterian Church but had rejected the idea of a God when, at the age of eleven, he watched his father die as a result of AIDS.

Drew had been such an easy child. Happy and fun, he loved his family, enjoyed his friends and enjoyed school. After two long years of trying to be the strength of the family by keeping his grief in check, Drew had slowly descended into a rough adolescence. He suffered from clinical depression, experimented with illegal drugs, separated himself from his family and his friends, and spent the next years in both a mental and spiritual isolation.

Upon graduation from high school and two years at community college, he enrolled in Texas Tech University in Lubbock. After reading Hemingway's *The Sun Also Rises*, Drew, in a search for something beautiful, decided to study abroad in Seville, Spain. His life was transformed by his time in Europe. Not only did he find people with whom he wanted to enjoy a real friendship, he also felt a spiritual awakening. He came home a changed young man and began reading everything he could about faith. After a year of personal study and prayer, he had chosen to convert to Catholicism. This weekend marked the culmination of his studies and his commitment to the Catholic Church.

Drew and I had lunch, and he was driving me back to my hotel so he could go to confirmation practice. Thinking about how far he had come, I commented, "You know, I was asked one time if I thought you would ever come back to the Church. Drawing my strength from God, I remember responding that I could see you back in the church one day, and although I didn't know how long it would take, I knew you would find your faith again."

His face deep in contemplation but with light shining through his eyes, Drew responded, "Can you believe this, Momma? Can you believe I'm being confirmed in the church tomorrow? It's hard to describe what I'm feeling. I'm almost giddy. I don't know. It's almost like I've been in the dark for the last fourteen years and this confirmation . . . somehow I feel like tomorrow is just going to wipe away those years, like I'm coming out into the light."

My eyes filled with tears as I thought about all that had happened in those fourteen years. We had traveled a journey that began with pain and loss, anger and disappointment. But has resulted in change and growth, accomplishment and redemption. It was a triumph over a journey that began with the ringing of a telephone.

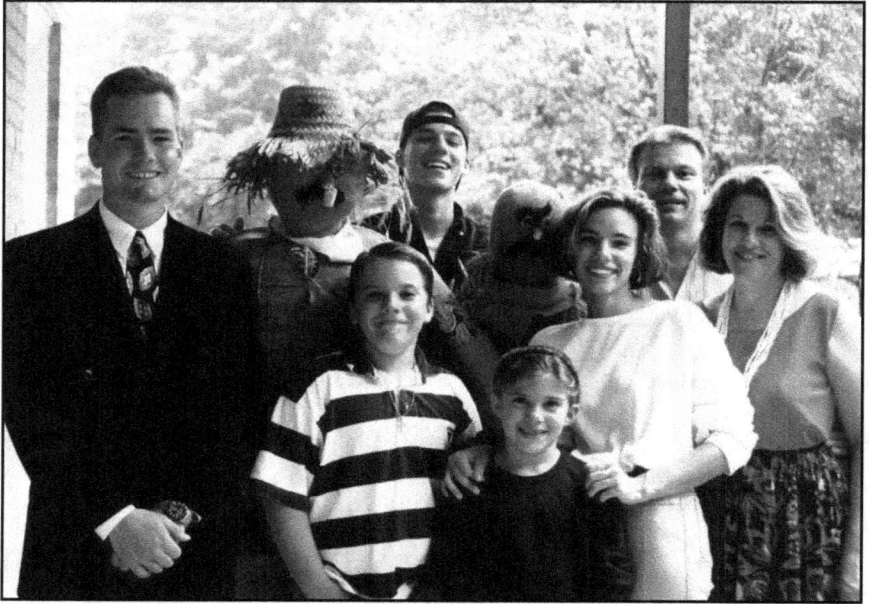

The Curtis family (from left to right)
William, Drew, Samuel (back row), Elizabeth, Kathryn, Dennis (back row), Joan

CHAPTER 1

The Beginning— December 1993

We are forty-three years old, married twenty-two years, and have five children. William, whom we adopted at the age of eighteen, is now twenty-one, Kathryn is nineteen, Samuel is fifteen, Drew is ten, and our baby, Elizabeth, is six. I have been a stay-at-home mom for most of our married life but have begun working this year at the small school Drew and Elizabeth attend. Dennis is an accountant by education, but he has had his hand in various endeavors. He developed accounting software in the late 70's and early 80's for small businesses; he ran an outpatient rehabilitation center; he opened a small medical clinic, "a doc-in-the-box" type of facility in 1990. Ever the entrepreneur,

Dennis is always right on the forefront of what is about to be big, but he never has the capital necessary for a lasting success. When the medical clinic failed, he had a difficult time coping with what he saw as his failure to provide adequately for his family. He is now involved in the service business but wants to go to Virginia to open a new office. We have stopped our medical insurance to save money for a new business, and Dennis has let his life insurance lapse as well. As we've talked about the need to go somewhere else to make contacts and the opportunities that Northern Virginia offers because of its proximity to Washington, I've spent several weeks thinking about all the aspects of a possible move. Right after Christmas, Dennis and I sit down, and I tell him my thoughts about the move.

"I think you should go to Virginia and make your contacts. I understand the importance of that piece, the networking, and even support your endeavor. But I don't know if this company will make it; we've seen some grow and others fail, and I'm not willing to uproot Drew and Elizabeth by taking them out of school in the middle of the year. Plus, I really like my job at Good Shepherd and don't want to leave it. How does this sound—you go and take Samuel and William? Samuel is not happy here, and he can get a fresh start in a new school there. William can get a job and help you or enroll in school. He's twenty-one years old so let him decide where he wants to put his efforts. Kathryn will finish the semester at the university in Ohio, and then she can join us in Virginia for the summer. Drew, Elizabeth, and I will finish the year at Good Shepherd. Drew is having a great year in fourth grade with Miss Dorsey, and he loves his soccer team. Elizabeth loves her first grade class, and I just can't disrupt all that. If the company is up and running by summer, then I'll start making the arrangements to move. Why don't you plan to leave early in January? By then, Samuel will be finished with his semester exams so he will be at the beginning of a new term when you get there."

Dennis agrees with my thinking, and we begin to plan for the move despite a rough couple of weeks in December with Dennis in bed with the flu. Samuel takes his exams in early January, and the next week, the three older men in my life leave for Northern Virginia. I take the day off from work and walk around the house wondering if Dennis will be able to pull this new company into the ranks of profitability. I also wonder if all the laughter has left the house because Samuel and his dad tend to keep me laughing.

It doesn't take long for Drew, Elizabeth, and me to adjust to a house of three. We enjoy our time together, like that our paths cross at school, and that we all ride home together at the end of the day. Drew plays basketball and soccer on the school team, so our entertainment is going to his games.

In February, the afterschool program where I work decides to put on a talent show. The students develop their own acts, and I decide Drew, Elizabeth, and I will sing a song together. None of us are musically inclined, but this is all for fun, so they agree without too much resistance. I choose a song that seems to represent the three of us in spirit since our husband and father, daughter and sister, and sons and brothers are all far away from us. On stage, Drew, Elizabeth, and I sing an off-key rendition of "Side by Side" without any premonition of future events in our lives.

"Oh, we ain't got a barrel of money. Maybe we're ragged and funny. But we'll travel along, singin' a song, side by side. We don't know what's comin' tomorrow. Maybe it's trouble and sorrow. But we'll travel along, singin' a song, side by side."

It is two months after Dennis, William, and Samuel have left for Virginia. They have settled into an apartment, and Samuel is in school, but Dennis is sick. A relapse of the flu he had in December has kept him from making any headway with his work, and he cannot seem to "kick it" this time. At 8:15 a.m. on Monday, March 14, the phone rings. I jump out of the shower to grab the receiver and hear a barely audible, "Scott, help."

"Dennis, is that you?"

"It's me." Again, barely loud enough to hear.

"Are you okay? Honey, what's wrong?"

"I'm sick; I need help, Scott. I need help."

"Okay, okay. What do you want me to do? Do you want me to come there?"

"Yes, come. Please come. Please help me, Scott." I can hear the choked-back tears.

"Okay, I'm hanging up to make a reservation and call Good Shepherd. I'll call you back as soon as I know the details. I love you, Dennis, so just hold on; I'm coming. Don't worry, Honey, I'll be there as soon as I can, and I'll take care of you. It's going to be okay."

I think about how Dennis has always called me by my maiden name, never by my given name as I catch a flight later that morning and fly into Washington, D.C. It's too late to go to the doctor, but I am able to make an appointment for the next morning. We get there early and within fifteen minutes, they are directing me to take Dennis to Fairfax County Hospital because he has pneumonia in both lungs. When he doesn't respond to any kind of treatment by that evening, the doctors request permission to test for HIV. We laugh—we've been married twenty-two years and have been together for twenty-three years—HIV is not a concern. We give permission.

That night, Mary calls to check on Dennis and on me. Mary, a dear friend from home, is the principal of the high school that Kathryn and William attended, and she and I got to be good friends because I did so much volunteer work at the school. I tell her the latest news, that his pneumonia is not getting better, and they have requested permission to test for HIV. "Wouldn't that be a kick in the butt if he has HIV?" I ask Mary rhetorically.

On the morning of Thursday, March 17, a doctor I have not seen walks with a nurse into Dennis' room. "Excuse me, Mrs. Curtis, but we need to speak to Mr. Curtis alone. The nurse will show you to a waiting area."

The nurse motions toward the door, and we leave the room. My mind is in fast forward. *Why would they ask to speak to him alone when we've been married twenty-two years? Oh my gosh, could he be infected with HIV? Is that why they want to talk to him without me? I know this is a crazy thought, but they did ask to test him for HIV on Tuesday and what else would require private conversation?* Calm down, Joan. Don't panic until you have a reason to panic. All of these thoughts zoom through my brain within the first minute of the three minute walk to the waiting area.

I am not there long. The nurse returns shortly and escorts me back to the room. The doctor leaves the room, and the nurse busies herself at the sink area. Dennis begins, "I have good news and bad news. Which do you want first?"

"You know me, Dennis. Give me the bad news and let me end with the good."

"The bad news is I have AIDS. The good news is I am getting over the pneumonia." Calm and matter-of-fact. No drama. Here it is, the kind of news that will change my and my family's life forever. I try to remember to breathe and wonder if I need to make sure my heart is beating.

The nurse asks me if I am okay and opens the door to signal the doctor to return. The doctor, a specialist in infectious diseases, explains that because Dennis' CD4 count is so low, he has probably been infected for about thirteen years. "The average healthy person has a little over a thousand T cells, and once infected, the virus destroys fifty to one hundred a year. What were you doing thirteen years ago?"

"Taking care of my brother who had been critically brain damaged in a car accident," I respond. My older brother was in a car accident, and he came to live with us for awhile.

"Did he have any blood transfusions at the time of the accident, and where is he now? What year was this?"

"The accident was in 1981 and yes, he had more than fifty units of blood given to him in the county hospital in Houston, Texas. He died in 1983."

"You and Dennis took care of him? How?"

"Scotty, my brother, was thirty-six years old when he had his accident. He was in the hospital and rehabilitation center for eight months before they released him for psychological reasons. His doctors said he needed to get out of the institutional environment. My parents were having a really difficult time coping with what had happened, so Dennis and I said he could come live with us for awhile. And actually, Scotty coming to our house was Dennis' idea. He has spent his life taking care of everyone else. Anyway, we had fulltime nurses, but Scotty wanted Dennis to do some things, and Dennis didn't mind."

"So, did he ever get body fluids from your brother?"

"Yes, the one time I'll never forget is when Scotty's plumb button came out, and Dennis tried to reinsert it. Scotty had a tracheotomy to ease breathing and had a plumb button to keep the opening from closing but protected to reduce risk of infection. One evening, that button just popped out, and I panicked because I was afraid the opening would close, and Scotty would die. Dennis, always calm, tried to put the button back in the opening and got blood all over his hands. He couldn't do it, and we had to take Scotty to the emergency room."

"Okay, well, let's just deal with what we have now. Dennis, you have almost no immune system left. We'll start you on AZT immediately as well as continue to treat the pneumonia."

AZT is an antiretroviral drug used for the treatment of HIV/AIDs. First approved for treatment of HIV, it was a major breakthrough in AIDS therapy in the 1990s that significantly altered the course of the illness. It also helped destroy the notion that HIV/AIDS was an instant death sentence. AZT slows HIV spread significantly but does not stop it entirely.

"Joan, I'm not going to give you any false hope," the doctor said matter-of-factly. "There is a slight chance that you won't be infected, but it is only slight. Dennis has been infected for a long time. Were any of your children born in the last thirteen years?"

"Yes, Drew is ten and Elizabeth is six. You're not saying ..."

"I'm not saying anything yet. If they've always been healthy, that's a good sign. Right now, let's get you to the lab and have you tested. Then we'll see where we are."

The nurse, once again, is my escort. She asks if I have questions, but I ask nothing. Thoughts are flying through my head. *AIDS! He has AIDS! Okay, okay, calm down, Joan. Think, don't panic yet. You don't know everything yet. AIDS! He has AIDS, and Dr. Wesley said thirteen years. He's been infected for thirteen years; how could I not be infected? Calm down, just think calmly, don't panic now. AIDS, my gosh, we don't even have medical insurance now; what were we thinking? Thirteen years! 1981! Before they knew anything. Drew and Elizabeth were born after that. My god, Joan, how are you going to tell Kathryn and Samuel and William that they're going to lose everyone? God, how? Don't think, Joan. Keep moving and don't think.* I take the first of many deep breaths.

CHAPTER 2

Miracles Still Happen—
Tuesday, March 22, 1994,
8:15 a.m.

FAIRFAX COUNTY HOSPITAL LAB
RUSH TO: Northern Virginia Clinic of Infectious
Diseases
Date: *March 19, 1994* Patient: *Joan S. Curtis*
Tests: *HIV*   Results: *Negative*
Culture tested for presence of HIV antibodies. None
detected. Patient should be retested in 6 months.

I have called Dennis to tell him that I'm on my way, and Doctor Wesley has personally come over to give him the news. Dennis is so excited, he yells into the phone. "You're negative!" It is too much to absorb. He has AIDS, and I'm not infected. It is much too much to absorb.

Those First Decisions After the Diagnosis— Tuesday, March 22, 1994

Dennis and I spend the morning celebrating the miracle that I am not infected. We seem to forget that he has received a death sentence; we are all smiles because I haven't.

Later in the afternoon, I go to the office of Dr. Wesley, the infectious disease specialist. I tell him about our family and our life in Dallas built over twenty-three years and now Dennis' desire to move to Northern Virginia to begin again. "Are you sure I'm negative, and, if so, how do you explain it?"

"Yes, you are negative. At least, you test negative now. Although when the virus first enters the body, the antibodies do not show up immediately. You can get a false negative, meaning you test negative even though the virus is present. That's why we recommend being retested in six months. You might be the one we hope for, the one who really is negative, the one we can never explain.

And if you test negative in six months, we don't need to test your younger children because they've always been healthy, and there's no reason to even suspect infection.

"Regarding your question about moving here or taking Dennis back home, you have to decide that for yourself. But I will tell you that ninety percent of fighting AIDS is mental—maintaining a positive mental attitude. If by moving here, you show Dennis that you believe in him and his ability to build this company, then that gives him a reason to get well and keep moving forward. On the other hand, if he goes back to Dallas and sees that as failure on his part to get this company up and going, it will be easier for him to give up on everything. That's what you have to be afraid of, his giving up. When I say ninety percent of the fight against AIDS is attitude, I don't want to make it sound easy. It is hard, damn hard—it's expensive, involves several medications, periodic illnesses—and that's the best case scenario. By the time you get to the diagnosis of AIDS, there is little of the immune system left—less than two-hundred T-cells. Dennis only has a fourth of that number, meaning he has little to nothing to fight off infection. So if you decide to move here, you have to do that now, not wait until summer. Dennis needs you now. The pneumonia is taking its toll, and it's going to be some time before he feels good again. Joan, Dennis has been given a time bomb for his life, and he needs you to help keep the ticking in the background and in check. Right now you have one fear—his giving up.

"I know this places a huge burden on you, Joan. I'm going to ask you a question and hope you don't take offense. Are you a woman of faith?"

"Yes, I am. I am a Christian, and my faith is the very center of who I am."

"Ironically, the two places that people with AIDS needed to be able to turn to for shelter in the beginning of this epidemic were two entities who were the most vocal about shutting them out—the family and the church. Some churches have finally turned around and have been a haven for people with AIDS, and one of those churches is the Episcopal Church. It's funny, really, because even the Episcopal Church is split right down the middle: either the local church is totally with you or totally against you. We have a local church here that fits into the first category. Would you like to go out and talk with someone there?"

"That would be good. That would be more than good." I've managed to keep it together for most of the day, but now the tears are starting to fall.

Dr. Wesley hands me a card. "Ask for Dr. Jerry Wilkinson. I'll call him and tell him that you are coming."

I look at the card. *Episcopal Church of the Good Shepherd. A Christ Centered Community. 9350 Braddock Road, Burke, Virginia.* My heart stops for a minute—Episcopal Church of the

Good Shepherd in Virginia, Good Shepherd Episcopal Church in Dallas—*God, You are in this, and You're letting me know. I am not alone. I will get my strength from You, God, for this journey.*

As I drive to the church, I think about all that Dr. Wesley has said. This is a most difficult decision because it means taking Drew and Elizabeth away from all they know, and it means leaving my friends, too. My mind wanders to the spring of 1971.

Dennis and I met the one semester we both attended Kilgore College in Kilgore, Texas. It was a community college, and several people from our hometown of Longview were taking classes also. About eight people met at the library between classes, and Dennis and I were among the eight. In April, he asked me to a concert in Shreveport, Louisiana, about an hour's drive from Longview. We didn't have another date until the middle of June, and that was really the beginning of us.

The oldest of four children, Dennis' mother had gone through three husbands and was on the fourth by the time we met. Dennis had assumed responsibility for the well-being of his younger siblings because he felt his mother seemed to put the men before her children. Dennis always described their childhood as one to be seen and not heard and always clean. "We were expected to play outside and not ever get dirty," he had told me more than once. "Looking and acting perfect, that is what she wanted from us."

Dennis never planned to marry because he didn't want to be responsible for more people, but we both felt something almost immediately. Accustomed to taking care of other people, he took me everywhere I wanted to go, which was something lacking in my previous relationship. He listened to what I said, played the music I wanted to hear, and never failed to call as soon as he returned from his off-shore drilling job in South Louisiana. We married the next summer, and he went to work so I could finish school first. We had our first child right after I graduated, and he couldn't have loved her more. With each of our children, he fell in love all over again. And when he saw the opportunity to save eighteen-year-old William from an abusive home life, he jumped at the chance to do for William what he had spent his childhood waiting for someone to do for him.

Remembering how few people Dennis had ever felt really loved him, I know what I have to do. I need him to believe in himself because he knows I believe in him. We have to move to Virginia, and I would figure out how to make it work for everyone.

Later that evening at the hospital, Dennis and I have come to the conclusion that we have nothing to hide concerning his having AIDS so we will be open and honest about this diagnosis. We know it will be easier if we're not trying to keep a secret. This is 1994, not 1984; we can talk about AIDS; people are smarter now. We are comfortable with our decision, and that we have decided something. Deciding something is better than sitting in the middle of a "maybe."

The 10 o'clock news begins. "Today in Fairfax, an ambulance was called for an extremely ill young man. However, family members report that when the ambulance arrived and the paramedics learned the patient had AIDS, the paramedics refused to transport the man. Further details later in the newscast."

Thoughts race through my head again. *Elizabeth is in first grade. Is that what will happen? You can't play with Elizabeth anymore; they have AIDS in their house. And what about Drew? We can't tell a ten year-old that his father is dying, and then tell the same child he can't talk about his father's illness.*

Dennis is thinking the same thing so within minutes we have decided not to tell anyone. We can't because Dennis is going to get better, and our first priority is to protect our children.

Dennis' lungs have cleared up enough by the end of March that he is discharged on Thursday, March 31. Dr. Wesley gives him three prescriptions, two for the pneumonia and one for AZT to fight the virus. We stop by the bank and withdraw six-hundred dollars to cover the medications and to buy Kathryn's plane ticket home. She is flying home for spring break. We plan to go by the airport after we get the medicine. We stop by a drug store and have the prescriptions filled. Each one is for one month, enough to get us home to Dallas and back to Virginia. The pharmacy bill is $586.58; that leaves us thirteen dollars and some change to pay for the plane ticket. Another reality of AIDS is beginning to take form. How are we going to do this? How?

Can I turn this over to God? I know I can, but the thought scares me because I think I need to have some control. And that's the thing—I think I need to be in control, but, really, I know I have no control. What I can do is continue to move forward and trust that I can continue to draw my strength from God. I will not hesitate to ask for His help. Help me, God, help me. This is in Your Hands.

CHAPTER 3

The Truth and the Whole Truth

We spend a few more days in Virginia because Dennis has some recuperating to do before he travels, and we need to find a place to live when we return. Dennis, William, and Samuel have been living in an apartment, but an apartment is not going to hold a house full of furniture. I stay with Dennis while William looks at houses with an agent. Once we settle on one, we meet with the leasing agent, sign the lease, give him six months rent, and make plans to return to Texas. We have not said anything to the kids, but the time is coming; we have to tell them something. The thought of lying to them makes me nauseated, but protecting them from what other people might say is the overriding thought.

Once we get home, we begin the process of deciding what to tell our family and our closest friends. That is how I have come to accept what I have to do. There is the truth and the whole truth. The truth is that Dennis is critically ill, and we need to move to Virginia where they are doing research related to his lung problems. The whole truth is that Dennis has AIDS, and we're moving to Virginia because that is what I've come to believe is the only thing that will prolong his life—my belief in him.

We know we have to tell our kids before anyone else so we stay silent and wait until Kathryn comes home for spring break. On Sunday, we call a family meeting, and everyone is wondering who is in trouble. The words do not come easily. Daddy has a disease—no name—and it is incurable. There is medicine, which treats the symptoms, but he will die eventually, and we have no idea how long, but it will not be anytime soon. Northern Virginia is a hotspot for research for this lung problem so we are moving to McLean, Virginia, in two weeks. Elizabeth is six, and Drew is ten; they are trying to figure out what we are saying. Samuel, fifteen, gets up and walks out of the house, and Kathryn, nineteen, runs after him. William, twenty-one, asks question after question; none of which really get answered. Somehow the minutes keep ticking away, and the day finally ends.

Now we move on to the others. Family— Dennis does not want any of his family to know so they get only the truth, incurable disease with no name. I know that I have to have my sister Judy with me on this journey, but I cannot tell her on the phone. She not only loves me, she adores Dennis, and this news will break her heart. I call her and tell her that I am flying to New Orleans to see our ninety-three-year-old grandmother and stopping in Houston on the way because I need to talk to her. She meets me in Hobby Airport, and somehow I put words together to make a sentence that includes Dennis and AIDS and no immune system and Virginia. We hug and hold each other for what seems like a lifetime. As I walk to the plane, I look back to see Judy staring at me, tears running down her face.

I do not even mentally debate about whether to tell Mother. Probably for thirty-five of my forty-three years, I have been taking care of my mother, and I just do not have it in me to take care of her right now. I arrange to meet Mother in Canton, halfway between her home in Longview and mine in Dallas. Over lunch, I tell her what we have told the children and Dennis' family—lung problems, incurable, research, moving. Mother drives home in a state of disbelief after I assure her that I will be okay. Of course, I will be okay; I am Joanie; I am always okay.

The friends who are told the whole truth can be counted on one hand—Alice, Becky, and Nancy. These are women who have been friends of mine for the majority of the time I've lived in Dallas. I met Alice in 1980 at church. Becky, too, I met at church in 1987. Nancy lives in the neighborhood, and we have been walking buddies for several years. I take assurance in the fact that they are all women of faith and will never betray my trust. When I go to Good Shepherd to quit my job, Headmistress Victoria Albright somehow has the words that draw the whole truth from me. Her tears mix with mine as she holds me close. Next thing I know, Victoria is handing me a check for the year's tuition for Drew and Elizabeth. "I know you're going to need this. It can help with the move."

Okay, we have told everyone what we can tell them. Now the packing starts—sixteen years in the same house and the dismantling begins.

Kathryn flies back to Oxford, Ohio, where she is completing her sophomore year at Miami University. Drew and Elizabeth go back to Good Shepherd for two more weeks. Mostly, we continue on as if nothing has changed—except everything in our house is being put into boxes, and I'm going out for lunch almost every day to tell someone else good-bye.

Dennis' sister, Margaret, has worked for Dennis for the past twelve or thirteen years, and she comes over every day to pack. I make little contribution. I am operating in a fog. No one really sees it, but I know I am on automatic pilot. I have to wear a mask. I am with people who know me, and they cannot see past what they have been told about Dennis. He is still not well enough to do much. We would be getting nowhere if Margaret was not helping us with this.

I wake each morning, but I wake with questions. What is happening? I look around and see everyone and everything familiar, but each moment feels surreal. I know I cannot keep going unless I find someone to talk to, and I have to know that this person will keep our conversation in confidence. I also have to know that I won't be facing judgment when I say the word *AIDS*. I find this person in Louise "Bo" Farrier at my Dallas church, Preston Hollow Presbyterian. Bo is an interim pastor, in place while we search for the right person. She welcomes me into her office, and within five minutes, she knows the most important information—AIDS, moving, five children, housewife. She has never seen me before this meeting, and she is crying within three minutes. Moving closer to me, she grasps both my hands and begins praying aloud. I don't really hear her, but her touch calms my heart. I stay with her for about forty-five minutes and leave knowing that God will give me the strength that I need. I don't have clarity yet, but at least my mind is quiet now.

There is really no money to hire movers, so we contract with U-Haul for the largest truck they have. I am trying to picture myself driving this truck when the first angel appears. John Fowler, the husband of my dear friend Nancy shows up at the back door one day. "Joan, I'd like to drive the truck to Virginia, if you don't mind."

"John, that's too much, but thank you. We'll figure it out."

"No, Joan, you'll be doing me a favor, honestly. First, I drove a truck years ago so this will be fun. Second, I was stationed in Northern Virginia and still have several buddies there. I really want to see them and revisit the base, and this is the perfect opportunity. I'd say you could pay me by buying a ticket to fly back, but since Nancy works for American, we've got passes that we haven't even used." He takes my hands in his. "Joan, please let me do this."

It is all I can do not to throw my arms around his neck and say thank you, thank you, thank you. Instead, very calmly the words come, "Okay, John, thank you. That really will help. Do you have any specific time frame of having to be back?"

"I actually have several weeks free so if I'm back by the end of April, I'm good."

"Okay, we have tentatively scheduled the truck for pick-up on April 12, but we do want the kids to finish that week of school. We thought we'd get them after school on that Friday and drive part of the way."

"If I leave on the thirteenth, that gives me two or three days start on you all, which is what we want. It would be best if I could drive straight to the house."

Funny, it's my life, but John has thought of things that I haven't even considered. Again I wonder, how are we going to do this? "Alright, I'll call U-Haul and make arrangements to get the truck on the eleventh. I have hired three young men to pack the truck so I'll call them today to make sure they can be here early on the twelfth. We'll pick up the kids from school on the fifteenth and meet you in McLean on the seventeenth. I'll get the address and phone numbers to you before you leave."

The days pass; John leaves in the truck on Tuesday, and the fifteenth arrives like any other day. My dear friend Alice calls early in the morning to tell me that her mother has died. Her mother had been ill for some time, but I cannot believe she is gone on this day, the day we leave. Alice and I make plans to meet for lunch at 11:30 at Preston/Royal.

"Joan, do not even think about postponing leaving here."

"But, Alice, if the service is tomorrow, I can be there for you, and we can leave right after that."

"No, Joan, don't do that. The service is to-morrow, but you can't put the kids on hold. Psychologically and emotionally, you have to leave with them today, just as you've planned. That's only fair to them."

I know she's right, but my heart hurts so much for her and for me. I loved her mother. "I know we should go; it's going to be hard enough as it is. Just know that I am with you tomorrow. I wish I could stay longer and talk, but I do have a few last minute errands. I took film to the Sam's Club on Beltline and need to pick up the pictures before we get the kids."

"I am coming up in October whenever our fair week-end is," Alice begins to choke.

"Remember we're not going to cry. We'll see each other soon; it'll just be longer between lunches." I am choking back tears, too. Thoughts race through my mind. Alice and I have been friends for fourteen years. She kept the boys when my older brother Scotty died and again when Daddy died. Sometimes I think she knows me better than I know myself. How am I going to walk this journey with her so far away? We hug; we cry; we take one last look at each other; we get into our cars and drive away.

I go by the house to check on Dennis and then run to Sam's to pick up the pictures. It is out of the way, but I know they charge much less to develop pictures, and I know the money, even five or ten dollars, saved now will matter later. I park the car and jump out; it takes about 30 seconds for me to realize that I have locked the keys in the car. Do not cry, Joan; do not cry. If you start now, you might not stop. I go inside and get the pictures and call a locksmith. He is there in twenty minutes, and, fifty dollars later, I am on my way. No money saved with these pictures.

I pick up Dennis, and we leave Margaret there. She is going to go through the house one more time before locking it. For now, we have decided to just leave it vacant, and Margaret has agreed to check on it every week or so. We do not linger; this is too hard. Dennis and I drive to Good Shepherd, park, and wait for the bell to ring. In a few minutes, I see Elizabeth running toward the car and then Drew catches my eye. His face is resolute, but the sadness in his eyes pierces my very soul. He opens the door to the car. "Let's go. Let's just go." He closes the door.

Oh, God, what are we doing? If this is what I have to do for Dennis to live, okay, but am I breaking the kids in the same process? Get hold of yourself, Joan, it will be okay. You are going to make this work.

Drew and Elizabeth are buckled in; our dog Shishkabob is sitting quietly in the back of the suburban. William and Samuel are in Kathryn's Sunbird behind us. I remind myself of what Victoria Albright had asked me that day at Good Shepherd. "You're not running away, are you, Joan?"

I had assured Victoria, "No, we're not running away. We're running to a new business venture for Dennis that will help prolong his life. We're not running away; really, we're not." By saying it out loud, I am assuring myself, too.

No, we're not running from Texas; we're running to Virginia. We cross the state line. Good-bye, Texas.

CHAPTER 4

Welcome to Virginia— The Dogwood State

We arrive in Virginia on Saturday, April 16, in the middle of an incredibly beautiful spring. Pink and white flowers are clustered together on tree after tree. The sheer beauty is breathtaking, and tears fill my eyes as I take in the dogwood and cherry blossoms. *Thank You, God. I feel like this is for me, that you're telling me, "Joan, see the beauty; it is all around you."*

As we drive to the house we've rented, I am reminded of why I fell in love with Northern Virginia the first time we thought about moving here fifteen years ago—the multitude of trees, many of which are pine. Growing up in the piney woods of East Texas, I feel at home here.

This feels good, and I hear a quiet voice in my head. It's the right thing.

Suddenly, I see an armadillo crossing the road right in front of the car. Armadillos belong in Texas; I can't believe I'm seeing one my first day in Virginia. About four blocks from the house, I see a man and a woman walking along the street. Taking a closer look, I catch my breath. I know that couple from my church in Dallas. Harriet and Chuck Gibbs had moved here about three years ago because Chuck went to work for a firm in Washington, D.C. The thought that has been constant in my head is that I am starting over because I will know no one, and now we're moving into the same neighborhood in Virginia as people I know. Taking deep breaths, I relax—pine trees, armadillos, Chuck and Harriet—we are not in a strange place after all.

Samuel, Drew, and Elizabeth begin school, the boxes are all unpacked, and the days take on a routine as if we have always lived here.

Once a week, I take Dennis in for a lung treatment. It takes about an hour and the cost is a hundred dollars. This will help dissipate the fluid remaining in his lungs as well as offer some protection against future build-up. Pneumocystis pneumonia is a constant threat for anyone infected with HIV. By the middle of May, still weak and feeling poorly, he is discouraged and announces that he cannot fight this thing after all.

I react quickly, "What do you mean, you can't fight this? You have to fight. We moved to Virginia for you; you can't give up."

Quietly, in short spurts of breath, Dennis explains further, "I'm tired, Joan." Dennis has called me Scott all of our married life. When he says Joan, I know there is trouble. "Even breathing seems hard. At times. I don't… know…I just don't…think….I can do this…I need you to call Restland."

"Call Restland? You mean Restland Funeral Home, as in Dallas Restland? Why?"

He explains to me that Cora, his grandmother, is buried there. "She's the one person who loved me unselfishly, and I think I want to be buried where she is. You have to call them and find out where she is and how much a burial plot costs there."

With a louder voice, I try to keep from screaming, "Dennis, you can't do this to me now. I left my family, my friends, my job, pulled the kids away from their school and friends—you can't quit on us. You can't."

Through clenched teeth, he controls his response, "Scott, I'm tired. I'm dying." Dennis is walking away and does not sound tired; he sounds angry.

I follow and do not care if I am shouting, "Do you think I don't know that you're dying? God, what do you think all this moving is about? I know it; I get it. But you can't just think about you. We are a family, and we're all affected so you cannot give up."

"I'm the one who's dying, Scott, not you, not the kids. Me, only me. You may think you get it, but you don't because it's not you. Men—husbands, fathers—die every day and life goes on. Wives remarry and children call their step-father Daddy and hardly anyone misses a beat. You all will be fine, and I'll be dead. That's the truth."

"Have you not heard anything I've told you for the last twenty-three years? I love you; you are my life. Don't you dare think I'm not dying here, too. You may be the one who gets buried, but I'm the one who has to figure out how to keep living. I'm dying, Dennis; I'm dying with you."

We stand there, energy spent, emotionally depleted, tears falling. I take him in my arms, and we hold on to each other as if we draw life's breath from the other—because we do. He sits on the sofa, and I go find the Dallas phone book so I can call Restland.

That night, Kathryn comes home from school in Ohio. She plans to spend a couple of weeks with us before she goes to Dallas to work for the summer. Kathryn and Samuel have struggled since William's adoption because they have felt their dad abandoned them to give William attention. She called about two weeks ago to tell me that she cannot live with us in Virginia and deal with both William and her father's illness. She has contacted our principal friend, Mary Steere, and Mary has agreed to let Kathryn live with her in Dallas while Kathryn teaches swimming lessons. Because we moved after she went back to school at the end of spring break, she has never been to the house in Virginia. I have sent specific directions to get there since narrow, curvy roads are more difficult to navigate when a multitude of trees block the light from the moon and stars. Driving here at night makes me feel completely alone, so I want to help Kathryn avoid that feeling.

Expected about 8:00, she arrives a little after 10:00. Dropping her suitcase and purse on the floor, she immediately yells at me about being lost and scared.

"Didn't you follow the directions I sent?" It has been an exhausting day for me, and what I do not need is Kathryn screaming at me when I made it as easy as I could for her without driving to Ohio to get her.

"Yes, but I know how you are about right and left so I turned left when you said right because I figured you got it wrong, and it is so damn dark. I hate this place!"

Calmly, I take her in my arms. "I know I sometimes get directions mixed up so I made a trial run writing everything down right as I did it so I wouldn't make any mistakes. I'm sorry you got lost." Since this is Kathryn's first time to see the house, she doesn't even know where her room is. "Let me show you your room. I know you're tired."

I don't tell Kathryn about that day for me—that I have spent the morning calling about burial plots and funeral costs for her father. Instead, I reassure her that's she's home now and things will look better in the morning.

I am doing everything I can to keep life normal for Dennis and our children, but all my friends are in Dallas. It doesn't take too long for me to realize that I have to have some support to get through this new stage in my life. Friends have always been my lifeblood, and I have to start meeting people. When I think about the friends I have in Dallas, I realize that most of them are connected to Preston Hollow Presbyterian Church, which I joined in 1975. I know I need people of faith so I begin going to churches. One Sunday I call the First Presbyterian Church in Arlington and inquire about directions. It doesn't seem far so I decide that's where I'll visit next. Although I have always taken the kids to church with me, I do not take them today; I need this time alone.

Walking in the church, I am met by the pastor, Roxanna Atwood. As soon as I open my mouth, she asks if I'm the person from Texas who called earlier about directions. When I nod, she grabs the arm of another young woman. "Beth, this is Joan Scott, who recently moved here from Texas. Will you sit with her? This is her first time to visit our church. Joan, this is Beth." We sit down, the service begins. The Preparation for Worship, the Confession, the Reading of the Word and Sermon and Offering and then the last hymn begins—"Here I Am, Lord":

I, the Lord of wind and flame, I will tend the poor and lame.
I will set a feast for them; My hand will save.
Finest bread I will provide 'till their hearts are satisfied.
I will give my life for them. Whom shall I send?

Here I am, Lord. Is it I, Lord? I have heard you calling in the night.
I will go, Lord, if You lead me. I will hold Your people in my heart.

Tears are coming so fast and furious that I am finding it difficult to catch my breath. Poor Beth has no idea what's going on, and I just collapse on the pew seat. The service is over. Beth leaves. I sit; tears continue to fall. *You've called me? Me? I'm nobody. Here I am, Lord. Here I am.*

CHAPTER 5

The Appearance of an Ordinary Life

By mid-June Dennis has recovered from the pneumonia and is feeling good. Upon release from the hospital in March, he had been put on azidothymidine (AZT). He decides not to take the AZT anymore. "Scott, I feel good now, and the medicine just reminds me that I'm sick. I think I'll do better without it. You know, not think about being sick."

I remember Dr. Wesley's words, *ninety percent of the fight against AIDS is a positive attitude*; I don't argue. AIDS is a terminal diagnosis, and Dennis needs time to process the diagnosis. Dr. Wesley has told me that many people will not take the medication for the same reason that

Dennis doesn't want to take it—you feel good, and it's just a reminder that you're sick. With the passage of time, most people begin to accept the diagnosis, and they start taking whatever they need to prolong their lives. I do not argue with Dennis now; I only hope he accepts the diagnosis soon and gets back on the AZT.

We moved to Virginia knowing no one, and it seemed as if we would never be at home in this place. New schools, new soccer teams, new church and they were all full of strangers. However, each day became another until, finally, we had all made connections and carved out a place for ourselves.

Life is good right now. The kids have all adjusted and made friends. As a first grader, Elizabeth has not missed a step and enjoys afternoons playing with friends. The move has been more difficult for Drew, but he has made some friends and is also playing soccer, so life has taken on a regular beat for him again. Samuel has a girlfriend and is getting his credits in high school. We spend several days at the beach during the summer, and a friend of Drew's from Dallas is able to come up for a week.

Kathryn leaves to study in Luxembourg and Switzerland. She had asked me during the summer if she should stay home, but Dennis has insisted she go forward with her plans to study in Europe her junior year. We use more savings to finance her trip. He has always tried to give his children what he did not get during his own childhood. William is bartending in Washington, and enjoying the interaction with the people he meets.

School starts again, and I decide I need a job to keep my mind occupied and provide a little income. Dennis is trying to make contacts but is not having any luck, and we have no steady income. We are using savings to cover our daily expenses. I know I need to be there when Drew and Elizabeth come home from school so I find a part time job in a family law practice. The hours give me time to see the kids off to school and be back on the corner waiting when their bus brings them home. I don't take the job under false pretenses. I tell them during the interview that my husband is terminally ill, and that may affect my being present at work if he gets sick and needs me home. They hire me anyway. I do clerical work, which is not difficult but does require concentration and attention to detail, exactly what I need.

I have found a circle of women at church and meet with them once a week. The first night I met with this group and said my husband was terminally ill, Laura said she understood because she had lost a friend to AIDS five years ago. I am amazed that I have been led to this group and AIDS is mentioned. I don't feel safe enough yet to reveal my "other life," but I know I want to come back and share time with these women. Although these months in Virginia have given us a lot of family time, I really miss my friends, and maybe I will be able to form genuine friendships with women in this group.

Alice flies up for a weekend in October, and we have a marvelous day in Harper's Ferry, West Virginia. Because of its strategic location on the Baltimore and Ohio Railroad during the 1860's, Harper's Ferry was a major location for movement of both Confederate and Union troops. As a history teacher, Alice is intrigued by the rich history of this place, and we treasure our day in Harper's Ferry. Red and gold and orange leaves fill our vision as we drive through the mountains.

Later in October, I fly to New Orleans to meet Mother. My grandmother, Mama Bec, had died in June, and Mother and I will spend this time together to go through Mama Bec's house. We spend a week in New Orleans, and we then drive back to Texas in Mama Bec's car. Mother gives me her car to drive back to Virginia as we have sold Dennis' car for medical needs. As I drive back to Virginia alone, I call home to let them know where I'm stopping to spend the night. No one ever answers. By the second night with no answer, my imagination takes over. Dennis has passed out, and the kids have taken him to the hospital where he's in critical condition, and they're just hanging out at the hospital. When I find them all at home and in good shape, I'm almost mad. An active imagination can be a dangerous commodity.

Drew, Elizabeth, and I spend a November weekend in Virginia Beach for Drew's soccer tournament. We take a side trip to Colonial Williamsburg. I am fascinated by the buildings, the streets, the period clothing worn, but my children do not seem too interested in all the history of our surroundings. They do enjoy the time at the beach, and this soccer tournament being held at the beach allows for a couple of afternoons in the sand.

Another November Saturday finds Elizabeth and me driving down to Charlottesville, Virginia, to spend the day with my brother, Arthur, and his partner Dan. We pick apples, and Arthur shows us how they make the cider. He and Dan are both wonderful with Elizabeth, and I feel relaxed for the first time in a long time. That was a good day.

Our life in Virginia has taken on an appearance of normalcy. The kids go to school; I have a job; we have visitors and take little trips. No one knows that Dennis has AIDS. I go alone to the Elizabeth Taylor AIDS Clinic in Washington, D. C., for another HIV test. Again, I am negative. I have to wonder about God's plan for me. Dennis has been infected with that virus for thirteen years, but I didn't get it. This is a miracle. It's hard for me to think that. *Me? A recipient of a miracle? But what else can you call it? It is a miracle, so there must be a reason. What is God's plan for me? And how long will I have to lead two lives?*

Mother flies up for Thanksgiving and before it's over, Dennis begins to run a low-grade fever. His throat is bothering him, and he is diagnosed with thrush, a yeast infection leading to sores in the mouth and on the tongue. Neither is easy to cure because of his suppressed immune system. The bottoms of his feet are showing signs of neuropathy, an inflammation of the nerves, and hurt most of the time. He does not leave the house often. I finally feel like I can tell Mother the truth. I have to tell someone. I feel so alone. "Mom, I have to tell you about Dennis. It's more than a lung disease, which is why his throat and feet are bothering him now."

"Honey, what's wrong with him? I've been wondering why his feet were causing such problems." Mother is troubled by my news.

"Well, the kids don't know, but he has AIDS, and—"

"AIDS? How in the world did he get AIDS?"

"We don't know for sure, but the doctor said he'd been infected for thirteen years. We were taking care of Scotty thirteen years ago."

Alarmed, Mother asks, "Did Scotty have AIDS? I don't remember that."

"No, Mom," I explain. "We'll never know if Scotty might have gotten infected blood when he had his accident, but it does make sense. He died in 1983, and they hadn't even named HIV yet, I don't think." Tearfully, I continue, "I don't know if that's how Dennis was infected or if he did something that he's not telling me, but I'm not dwelling on how he got it; I'm just trying to figure out how to keep him alive."

Somehow Mother pulls herself together and takes me in her arms. "I'm here, Honey. I'll do whatever I can for you. Don't hesitate to ask; I'm here."

Dennis is declining, and the medication is so expensive. We stopped the lung treatments because he didn't need anymore once the pneumonia was gone. Now he has so many other problems, and we simply don't have enough money to cover both a doctor's visit and multiple medications. I've tried to talk to him about keeping Kathryn home after this first semester in Europe, but he won't hear of it. He is determined to give Kathryn an unforgettable experience even if it means a choice between medical help or a European experience. He loves our children so much.

I read in the paper about a research study in HIV/AIDS at Johns Hopkins in Baltimore. Participants in the study will receive free medication. We are running out of money, and Dennis needs medications. Because Baltimore is only fifty miles away from our house in McLean, I make an appointment.

We arrive early in the afternoon and are shown to the waiting area. This area is about the size of a large doctor's office, and there are windows on one side. There must be twenty-five chairs, and at least twelve of them are occupied. Most of the people sitting in this room are African-American and really thin. Two or three of them look emaciated. Scattered around the room are at least four of those red plastic containers in which to dispose of infectious needles and other supplies. There are two kinds of people in this room—those with AIDS and those without AIDS. I think I might be the only one in the second category.

Blood is taken; a few tests run; the good news is that Dennis does not have CMV retinitis, an AIDS-related eye disorder that results in floating spots, flashing lights, blind spots, and blurred vision. The bad news is that because he does not have CMV, he is not accepted into the study. Like every doctor I have met on this journey, this one at Johns Hopkins wants only to help Dennis so she gives him his medications at no cost. She then assures us that he will continue to get what he needs, and he can come in for his medical check-ups, also at no cost. She does not mention AZT; I guess we are past that point now.

Kathryn comes home for Christmas, and Dennis wants to celebrate as we always have— in a big way. Money is tight so we sell my suburban. I love that car. I try not to cry; I tell myself over and over that it is only a car. I have my mother's ten-year-old Oldsmobile, and we have Kathryn's Sunbird.

I loved that suburban.

Dennis and I buy a multitude of gifts for the kids and have a wonderful Christmas dinner. The day is perfect. Sometime that evening, Kathryn walks into the kitchen and finds her father on the floor. She screams and helps him up. He has fainted. He is going downhill. Kathryn leaves for Switzerland, and I still don't tell her the truth. I want to, but I have promised Dennis. We no longer agree about the older kids knowing the truth, but I am abiding by his wishes because he is the one who is sick. It is not getting easier to live part of my life in a secret world.

CHAPTER 6

Living with AIDS in 1995

Disbelief
    105^0 fevers for eight hours a day, weakness,
    snow drives for medical care
        Secrecy.

Disbelief
    Waking up in soaking sheets, weekly lung
    treatments, mouth sores
        Secrecy.

Disbelief
    Blood transfusions, isolation, kidney
    failure, liver failure, weight loss
        Secrecy.

Disbelief
>   Changing sheets, wondering, tears,
>   questioning
>   Secrecy.

Disbelief
>   Inexplicable pain, mental confusion,
>   freezing inside, more tears, and
>   Always, always secrecy.

We have been in Virginia for eight months, and by mid-January, Dennis is experiencing night sweats along with the foot pain and mouth sores. Fevers are no longer low-grade but sometimes as much as 105 degrees and several hours a day. He asks me if I want to go home. I can see that he's not going to build a business. I can see that he's getting sicker every day. In my mind, I equate going home with going home to die. I say no, I like Virginia, and I want to stay here. Just as I am playing mind games with myself, so are William and Samuel.

William goes to work every afternoon, and I pick him up at midnight. He never asks about his father, and I never bring it up in conversation. I know he must see the decline, but I do not ask.

On January 29, we celebrate Dennis' forty-fourth birthday. He is too sick to get out of bed. Elizabeth comes in and pleads, "Daddy, we have birthday presents and a cake for you. Don't you want to come see it and open your presents?" He struggles to get out of bed, but, for Elizabeth, he makes himself get up and goes into the dining room so we can sing Happy Birthday, and he can open his presents. He puts on a big smile for Elizabeth.

By the first of February, I have made a decision to talk to Samuel. I do not want to tell him the truth but feel he must be told his father is dying. We cannot pretend otherwise. Saturday night I walk downstairs to his room and sit on the bed. My heart is beating so fast, but I speak calmly, "I want to talk to you about your dad." Samuel is quiet. "I know you are at an age when you want to spend all your time with your friends, and your family is on hold until later after you graduate. You have to have noticed that your dad is getting sicker so you might want to think about spending time with him now because I don't think he'll be here later after you graduate."

Samuel looks up and protests, "But, Mom, that's just two years from now."

"I know."

"Are you saying he'll be dead in two years? Mom, Drew and Elizabeth are so little."

"I know." We sit in silence for several minutes. "Samuel, I love you."

"I know, Mom."

The next afternoon, Sunday, I am looking for Samuel but cannot find him. Kathryn's car is gone. Dennis and I know Samuel has taken it, but he has told no one that he is leaving or where he is going. Neither of us is happy with him but I do not connect what I have told him last night to his being gone. About five o'clock, the phone rings.

"May I speak to Mr. or Mrs. Curtis, please. This is Matt Walton."

"This is Joan Curtis, Mr. Walton." I know this is the father of one of Samuel's female friends.

In a carefully controlled voice, he continues, "We just found a note from Lynn. She and Allison have gone with Samuel to Texas because they're afraid he's going to kill himself. She says Mr. Curtis is dying, and Samuel doesn't want to watch him die. Do you have any idea where they might have gone?"

Calm, Joan. Calm.

"I don't, but I will call his friends in Dallas and try to find them. I am so sorry, Mr. Walton. I'll call as soon as I know anything." I don't say anything about Dennis' health, and we hang up. Dennis and I are livid. *What in the world is Samuel doing? I feel guilty. Did I tell him too much last night? Is that why he's doing this? Oh, God, what's next? What?*

About 9:00 p.m. the phone rings. I grab it,

and hear Samuel, in an obviously troubled voice, say, "Hello, Mom? Is that you?"

Frantic, I reply, "Yes, it's me. Where are you? What are you doing?"

"I'm in Dallas at Calli's," he concedes. "The girls have called their parents, and they're gonna fly home tonight. I've already taken them to the airport. I just couldn't stay there and watch Dad get sicker. I just couldn't."

"So instead you leave without telling us and make us worry because we don't know where you are? Did you think that would help, Samuel?" I am angry and annoyed. "Did you think that would make everything okay? And getting Lynn and Allison to go with you so now their parents are mad at us? Did you think that was a smart idea?"

Now enraged, Samuel blurts out, "I already said I couldn't stay and watch Dad get sicker. I don't even like you all right now."

His words infuriate me so I bark back at him,

"Well, I can't say I like you very much right now either. You stay at Calli's, Samuel, because I am coming to Dallas." Slamming down the phone, I look at Dennis, "Now what?"

We decide I will fly to Dallas and get Samuel and drive him home. Alice will meet me at the airport, and I'll spend the night with her. I let my boss know that I'll be away from work for a few days.

By the time I get to Dallas, the girls have flown back to their parents, and Samuel has started driving back to Virginia. I call Dennis to see what we do next.

"You stay there, Scott. I'm okay for awhile. Samuel will get home later tomorrow, and I can take care of everyone. You spend a few days in Dallas with your friends. Get some rest. If you go down, we all go down. I can take care of things here. I love you, Scott; don't forget that."

Alice and I spend hours talking. It is so good to be with someone and not have to hide anything. I make plans with another friend, Annie, to go out to dinner and see a movie on Wednesday. Annie and Rob are the first couple friends we made in Dallas. Annie and I choose a new movie with Drew Barrymore, Mary Louise Parker, and Whoopi Goldberg, *Boys On the Side*. A movie about girlfriends and a road trip to Tucson; perfect. From the first indication that Mary Louise Parker's character is sick, I know it is AIDS. An hour passes before the illness is named in the movie, but I know. By the time the movie is over, both Annie and I are sobbing. I have to tell her that Dennis has AIDS. Neither of us can stop crying. By the time we get home and tell Rob what is going on, he's mad at me for getting Annie so upset. I leave feeling a little perplexed by his attitude. Does he not understand that Dennis is dying? I can't believe that he's that selfish, so I have to believe he really doesn't understand the gravity of what he's been told.

When I get back to Alice's, she tells me that Dennis has been calling. I return his call.

"Joan, you've got to come home. Samuel is really upset. He put his fist through the wall, and now Drew is upset because he's worried about Samuel. I can deal with Samuel, but I cannot take care of all three of them. You've got to come home and take care of Drew and Elizabeth."

"I'll make a reservation tonight and be home tomorrow. Just try to hold everything together until I get there." I don't have the money to fly home so Alice lends me the money for the ticket. I can't get a flight out until Friday. By the time I get home, Samuel has threatened to run away again, so Dennis has called the police and had Samuel taken to the juvenile center overnight. Dennis needs the rest and hopes maybe this will wake Samuel up.

Samuel comes home on Saturday morning just in time to stay with Drew and Elizabeth while I take Dennis to the emergency room at Johns Hopkins. Skin the color of gold, every movement he makes is laden with weariness. They admit him immediately; his liver is functioning at less than 20 percent. The ER nurse refers to him as *our golden boy*. I take the kids to see him on Sunday. By Monday, the doctors know his kidneys are failing, too. His doctor hopes to reverse everything. I am driving fifty miles there and fifty miles back each day. Tuesday, I see the white flakes drift down as I drive to Baltimore. By the time I drive home, the ground is completely white. Wednesday, the roads are still clear enough to get to Baltimore so I go after getting Drew and Elizabeth on the bus. William does not work today and will be there when Drew and Elizabeth get home so I do not have to worry about getting back. Early in the afternoon, Samuel's school counselor calls to tell me that Samuel is threatening to run away again. I ask them to keep him there, and I leave Dennis to go back to McLean to get Samuel. Drew is at a friend's house, and I call to see if he can stay there for awhile. When Samuel and I get home, William launches into his brother as soon as we walk through the door. "What in the hell are you doing? Trying to kill Dad?"

Samuel explodes, "Me? Who do you think fucked up this family by barging into it?"

Red-faced and seething, William moves closer to Samuel and responds, "You stupid little shit, Dad wanted me to join this family because you were already such a screw up. Now you're pulling stunts like this and putting him in the hospital." I move between them—one hand on each of their chests to hold them apart.

Huddled in a corner terrified, Elizabeth is crying, "Make them stop, Mommy; make them stop."

"You all can't do this. You can't. William, you've got to leave for awhile until you both calm down. And don't you dare call your dad and tell him about this," I am adamant. "Go now. Go."

Overwhelmed by everything that is happening, I run to get Elizabeth. Pulling her into my arms, I want to tell her that it will all be okay, but it is not going to be okay, and so I cannot say it. Instead, I just hold her close and whisper over and over, "I love you, Sweet Pea. I love you."

Drew spends the night with his friend, and Elizabeth sleeps in my bed with me. As everything seems out-of-control, I am restless and get little sleep. Sometime in the wee hours of the morning, I hear the front door so I know William has come home. I feel guilty. I know I should not have sent him away, but I am frightened of what Samuel will do next. *Where is the instruction book for this situation, God? What am I supposed to do?*

Elizabeth and Samuel leave for school the next morning, and William stays locked in his room. Again, I drive to Baltimore in the snow, but this time in full knowledge that I cannot continue to travel this journey alone and in secret. I park the car and walk into Dennis' room. Arms open and rising toward me, I fall onto the bed and into his waiting arms. Tears streaming, I plead, "Take me home. Please take me home."

CHAPTER 7

Going Home

We are going home; the decision has been made. The move that was to be forever has lasted nine and one-half months. I am just two weeks away from the first anniversary of the day I heard the words that changed my life forever. "The bad news is I have AIDS." For almost a year I have been living two lives, but at least now, I am going home.

This decision to go is the easy part; the hard part is the 1001 things that have to be done before we can leave Virginia. We have to wait for Dennis to be discharged from the hospital; we have to notify the leasing company; we have to find a place to live in Dallas because we have leased our house there; we have to pack and there is no Margaret to help; we have exhausted our financial resources from selling the suburban, to giving up my engagement ring and diamond drop that was a wedding gift from Dennis. William comes to tell me that he has money from the grandfather he had before he became part of our family. Withdrawing the money, it is enough to get us home, into a house, and carry us for a couple of months, but I have to have a job, and we have to have medical insurance. We have to withdraw the kids from school here and make plans to enroll them in Dallas. Will Good Shepherd let Drew and Elizabeth come back as if they have been on a long weekend break? And what about Samuel? Where will he go to school? And Kathryn? She's studying in Switzerland and knows nothing that has gone on in Virginia. I have intentionally not told her so that her time in Europe is everything it can be without the burden of worrying. What will William do? Get another job? The kids. We have to tell the kids that we are going home, but

I don't know when because it all depends on when Dad gets discharged.

The first thing I do is call my friend Mary, principal of the high school from which Kathryn and Matt graduated. She had told me in January that if we'd come home, she would hire me to be a clerk in her office and that way we would have medical insurance for Dennis. Mary is delighted that we're coming and tells me that she will hold the clerk's position until I get there, and I can turn in an application and resume then. Job and insurance settled.

I call Alice and ask her to find a house for us to rent. Yes, we want somewhere in the northwest section of Dallas; we have always lived there. We discuss an amount for monthly rent. This is a huge task, but Alice doesn't care. She is just thankful that we're coming home. She tells me that she will enlist our friend, Annie, to help. She calls that evening to let me know that the two of them have already gone to work. It never even occurs to me that they won't find a place for us to live. Phone calls back and forth with Alice confirm a house has been found with an excellent elementary school within two blocks. The lease is faxed, signed, and returned, and Alice arranges to get the key. House settled. I am walking step by step by step and completely on faith.

Drew and Elizabeth are not sure how to react when I tell them that we're going home. I had told them that we were moving to Virginia permanently so Dad could get another business up and running. It had taken Drew awhile, but he's made friends, he's playing soccer; he and Elizabeth are both happy here. We've taken trips to Colonial Williamsburg, my brother's apple orchard, soccer tournaments in Virginia Beach and Durham, North Carolina. At least every couple of months, we have ridden the train into D.C. and visited one of the Smithsonian Museums. Elizabeth, William, and I celebrated the Fourth of July on the mall of our nation's capital. Now we're switching gears? What about Dad's business? And are they going back to Good Shepherd? I have no answers about Good Shepherd or when we will actually leave because we have to wait for Dad to get out of the hospital. But they do need to start packing; first, pack clothes and toys that they are not using. I remind them: we are going home; this is a good thing.

William and Samuel, still reeling from all that has happened in the past couple of weeks, appear resigned to whatever I say. Okay, we are moving back to Texas. When? I am not sure, but hopefully by the first of March so we do not have to pay another month's rent. I'll know more when Dad is discharged. Okay, what do you need? If you will each begin packing, and, please, do your best to get along with each other.

I go back to work after being off for two weeks due to family crises, and everyone gathers round to find out what has happened. At the time of the interview for this job, I told them that my husband is terminally ill, and I do not know how long I will be able to work if his health begins to decline more rapidly. I tell them Samuel ran away for a couple of days; Dennis went into kidney and liver failure and is in the hospital; we are moving back to Texas. Linda, one of the younger attorneys who is on a fast track moving forward, comments, "Joan, your husband really is seriously ill, isn't he?"

"Yes, remember I told you all that during the interview?"

"I guess I either didn't take you seriously or forgot because you are always so upbeat. Is he really terminal? As in, is he really going to die?" She is not being insensitive or rude; I hear in her question how difficult it is for her to witness a life that is rapidly changing directions.

"Yes, he is. Honestly, I didn't want to go back to Texas because I thought he would just give up if we did, but the last two weeks have taken their toll, and I need my family and friends."

She puts her arm around my shoulders, "My God, Joan, are you okay?"

I laugh. "No, I'm not okay. But I will be; ten years from now, wherever I am, I will be okay." I've only had this job since October, but it has become so much more than I thought it would be. Originally, this job provided some income as well as structured time so that I was not home brooding about an unknown future. But my hours here have been valuable in terms of accomplishing a job that is appreciated and of making connections with the people with whom I've worked. I know I will miss the people in the law firm and be forever grateful that I had this time with them. Somehow I find the words to let them know what they have become to me.

Dennis is discharged on Saturday, and planning and packing begin in earnest. We have exactly two weeks until March 1, so we set February 28 as our departure date. Drew and Elizabeth tell their friends, and the phone starts ringing with announcements of food coming for dinner. We may not have Aunt Margaret to do our packing, but the Chesterbrook Elementary fifth-grade soccer team feeds us every night.

I call Good Shepherd about Drew and Elizabeth, and Victoria Albright, Headmistress, assures me that they are welcome and teachers will know to expect them. She is not sure about next year, but tells me not to worry, one step at a time. Before we leave town, Samuel and I put in a mandatory court appearance due to a speeding ticket he got when he ran away to Texas. Thankfully, the judge listens to Samuel's explanation of his terminally ill father and this sixteen-year-old's desire to die first, so the judge doesn't lock Samuel up for the next five years. The judge does explain to Samuel that a desire to commit suicide does not give Samuel the right to endanger everyone else on the road. Samuel actually received two speeding tickets during that trip, just twenty-five miles apart. By the grace of God, the county line is between those twenty-five miles, and because this judge only knows about the ticket in his county, I get to take Samuel home with me instead of to juvenile jail for the next five years. He does have a suspended driver's license for six months, which seems a small price to pay.

The day we plan to leave, Dennis is not feeling well and decides he cannot travel with our dog, Shishkabob. He asks me to take her to the SPCA. I make an attempt to remind him that Drew and Elizabeth love that dog, but I can see it in his face; he is doing absolutely all he can do. Dennis and William rent a truck from U-Haul; they rent the largest truck and a trailer to pull. We hire men to pack on February 27, and I withdraw Drew, Elizabeth, and Samuel from school. I then leave Elizabeth on the porch in tears as I take Shishkabob to the SPCA. My heart is in such pain as I see her tears and know my only resource is my faith.

I turn off the radio and say my prayer out loud. *"God, I feel Your love for us even though I cannot understand what is happening. Please,*

please let sweet Elizabeth feel the love You have for her and somehow help her know that I am doing the best I can do."

When I return, the truck has filled up too quickly, and a quick phone call confirms my fear: the largest truck that specific location rented to Dennis is not the largest truck that U-Haul has. But it is too late to change course now. We leave the washer and dryer; they are over twenty years old anyway. Non-negotiables are packed. I make a quick decision; I leave my two rocking chairs; one my grandmother gave me when I was pregnant with Kathryn and the other Dennis gave me for my birthday nineteen years ago. Elizabeth's wooden rocking horse has to stay as well. All are awkward pieces to pack, and the doors will shut if we leave them.

The phone rings; the SPCA just wants to let me know that Shishkabab has been adopted. I breathe a silent prayer, *Thank You, God.* I look at the rockers and the rocking horse and remind myself that they are just things, just things.

Tears fall as I climb the stairs and walk out of the house. It's been a year of family and togetherness, but it is time to go home. Suddenly, I am struck with the realization that going home does not mean living happily ever after.

CHAPTER 8

Getting Settled Again

Pulling away from the house in McLean, William is driving the truck, Samuel is driving Kathryn's car with Dennis as his passenger, and I am driving my Mother's car with Drew and Elizabeth. Our plan is to get to Little Rock, Arkansas, this first day, spend the night there, and arrive in Dallas tomorrow. Because we are doing no sight-seeing or touring, I have not packed clean clothes. We'll drive, stop for gas and food, sleep in a t-shirt, get up and go. We can bathe and change when we get home.

The first place we stop for gas, William complains that he's not comfortable driving the truck. It is big; he's unsure of the load; he's unsure of changing lanes. He is just really nervous, and he doesn't like it. Dennis volunteers to take over, and I argue the point. He just got out of the hospital; he's recovering, not recovered; this is just the kind of thing he should not be doing.

I watch Dennis slowly get into the truck. This picture is such a contrast to the man I married. That man almost always displayed uncommon strength to carry everyone through whatever valley they were in. Now I see a man who is weak and scared and seems to be making snap decisions as if he is the only one to be considered. I expect William to jump in and say he can do it, but he doesn't. We leave the gas station with Dennis driving the truck; Samuel and William in Kathryn's car, while Drew and Elizabeth ride with me.

After a long day, we pull into the motel parking lot in North Little Rock, Arkansas. I immediately notice that I have begun my period and my jeans are soaked with blood. I cannot believe I have been sitting like that for hours and haven't noticed; worrying about Dennis driving the truck has been my primary thought and that, coupled with keeping life looking normal for Drew and Elizabeth, left little time to take note of my jeans. I have no clean jeans and no place to wash anything. Our suitcases were the first items on the truck so there is no way to get to them. Samuel runs to the drug store for me, and I wash my jeans out in the sink with hand soap and hang them up on the shower rod to dry. Matt, Samuel, Drew, and Elizabeth go get pizza for dinner while Dennis sleeps and I rest. They bring back dinner for us, and we settle in for the night.

Later, I close my eyes and whisper my last prayer of the day, *God, please take care of Dennis and give him strength to drive the rest of the way. Open the kids' hearts to everything good that is going on around us and with us, and, God, I know it's silly, but please let my jeans dry by morning.*

We awake to snow on March 2, 1995, in Little Rock, Arkansas. Luckily, it is not a heavy snow so the roads are clear; it just means a little colder with no jackets for anyone and slightly damp jeans on me. We eat breakfast and head for home.

Upon arrival in Dallas, we go straight to Alice's to get the directions and key to the house she found. Dennis is tired so I suggest he remain at Alice's to sleep while the rest of us go to see the house. Only about three miles from our former neighborhood, I know the area well, and we'll be close to Good Shepherd Episcopal School for Drew and Elizabeth, as well as Thomas Jefferson High School, where I'll be working. The high school that Samuel will attend, W.T. White, is just two blocks away from the house so he can walk. We couldn't be in a better place without being in our own home.

The size fits us to a tee, also. Drew and William can share a room, and Samuel can have the small room off the kitchen; he needs his own space right now. Kathryn's full-size bed will fit easily into the third bedroom so Elizabeth can sleep there, and she'll share the bed with her sister when Kathryn gets home from Europe. Not ideal, I know, but it won't be for long. Our landlord, knowing Dennis has a precarious health condition, has agreed to a month-by-month lease. I make plans to call our tenants in the morning to see if they will agree to find another house within the next few months. To get Dennis home, really home, is important to me.

With my profound thanks, Alice goes home to check on Dennis. We begin to take boxes of clothes out of the truck. After we hear from Alice that Dennis is still asleep, Samuel and William begin unloading the truck as I direct what goes in the house and where and what goes in the garage for now.

I make sure all the kids are busy with unpacking, and I leave to find something for dinner. I run by Alice's, but Dennis is still sound asleep. I really don't want to wake him; I know the drive completely depleted him. I ask Alice if he can stay. She gets a pillow, which I gently slip under his head, and a light blanket, which I put over him. He barely stirs. I kiss him lightly, rub my hand across his cheek, and go get hamburgers. Once home, we eat and make ourselves comfortable for our first night back home in Dallas, in Texas.

The next morning I call Alice to check on Dennis, and, learning he's awake, I head over to see how he's doing after a good night's sleep. He is up and although rested, I can tell the drive from Virginia really took its toll. Alice has insisted he eat something, and I am grateful because I know he would not have listened to me. We go home and spend the rest of the weekend getting settled.

On Monday, after getting Drew and Elizabeth enrolled and situated in their classes at Good Shepherd, Samuel and I go to W.T. White to enroll him in school. He will finish his sophomore year here, and we'll see where we are in the fall. When the admissions office realizes he is in the tenth grade, they ask him to come back after spring break, which is the following week. The TAAS test (Texas Assessment of Academic Skills) begins on Tuesday, and the tenth grade tests are the state assessments for which schools and districts are held accountable. These school officials do not want to take the chance on an out-of-state student messing up their scores. Samuel is thrilled; he has another two weeks' vacation from school. I then go to Thomas Jefferson, sign all the paperwork, and tell Mary I will start in the morning. She is delighted. She needs my help professionally, but, more importantly, she is happy that she is able to help us.

On Tuesday, leaving Dennis to take Drew and Elizabeth to Good Shepherd, I report to work at 7:00 a.m. at Thomas Jefferson. I have done much volunteer work in this place; both William and Kathryn graduated from this school, and I have served as the president of the drill team booster club and coordinator of college night, as well as just volunteering to help in the office at times. Many of the faculty members know me and are not surprised to see me behind the desk; they assume I'm doing more volunteer work. I am accepted into the fold with no hesitancy. It feels safe to be here.

Following spring break, Mary introduces me to Rebecca Swenson who has taken the place of the Distributive Education teacher whose mother is ill. Rebecca will finish the year, and part of the job is to run the DECA store during the lunch periods. Mary wants me to help Rebecca in the store because she is new. Within two or three days of working together, Rebecca and I have shared a couple of stories and become fast friends. When I have a mammogram, and the results come back as slightly abnormal, I cannot believe everything will be okay because I have a husband at home who is dying. Rebecca understands my tears and immediately wraps me in her arms. When students look at these two teachers hugging each other, Rebecca looks straight at them and says, "So what are you looking at? Teachers are people and can have problems and need friends to hug them, too." Rebecca doesn't know what is wrong with Dennis; no one does. She, like everyone else, only knows that he is terminally ill. It has been difficult to live with this secret of AIDS, and I don't know how much longer I can continue to lead two lives.

A couple of weeks later, I am walking out to the DECA store to meet Rebecca when Denise McCafferty, a young reading teacher, catches up with me. Thinking out loud, I take Denise by surprise. "So how do you tell a six-year-old that her father is dying? I mean, does a six-year-old really even understand death? I am Christian. I do believe in eternal life, but all I can think about is that for Elizabeth, her daddy is not going to be here. Period. Not here." Denise remains silent as we walk but takes her hand and gently squeezes the back of my neck. I know I have made her uncomfortable with my sudden questions about death, but my head had felt like it would burst with the unspoken thoughts.

Later that afternoon, Rebecca comes down to the office and asks to talk to me privately. "Joan, I don't know what is wrong with Dennis, but I have to tell you something. Denise McCafferty just asked me if he has AIDS."

Maintaining a masked face, I ask, "Why in the world would she ask you that?"

"Apparently, you said something to her about Dennis dying earlier today, so she asked one of her community mentors if he was really that sick and what was wrong. I guess the lady knows you and said, 'No one is really sure, but we think he has AIDS, so you better stay away from the whole family.'"

I can't help it—the tears come. Now I know I cannot tell anyone the truth because the fear and ignorance still permeate every circle. Denise's community mentor has been a friend of mine for years; we used to walk together every day. My heart hurts. Really hurts. I take a chance, "Rebecca, Dennis does have AIDS, but I am not infected. That's the truth."

"Joan, my mother committed suicide when I was eighteen so I am petrified of having a baby and doing the same thing to her. Now we both know a secret and are sworn to silence."

I am reminded of a column Ellen Goodman wrote for the *Boston Globe* years ago about the difference in men's and women's friendships. Men are buddies because they've done something together—played on a team, fought in a war, played any kind of sport like tennis or golf. Women are friends because they've shared a deep secret with one another. That's what Rebecca and I have just done. She has let me know that she is my friend, and my secret is safe. I smile. I now have someone at school; my head won't burst.

CHAPTER 9

The New Normal

"You look great!" is a compliment that often accompanies noticeable weight loss. But, on occasion, noticeable weight loss is a sign of something sinister. Dennis is losing weight daily, has no strength or energy, and hasn't seen a doctor in two months. There just isn't any money.

For that reason, I am impatient to get our insurance in place. Two weeks after I begin my job, I receive a letter from human resources. In a nutshell, I learn that Dallas ISD takes the insurance premium out of the employee check in the month preceding the insurance start date, but does not pay the employee until the second month of employment. Quickly, I realize that I will not be able to take Dennis to the doctor until May because I will not get paid until April, and that's when they'll take out the first month's premium. I panic! With furrowed brow and a heart beating too fast, I hand Mary the notice.

"Call human resources and tell them that you've just moved here and need to get your young children to the doctor. Don't tell them about Dennis. Suggest that they take two months of premiums out of your April check, so that the start date is April first instead of May first."

I get HR on the phone, and they agree. I breathe a sigh of relief, and call the doctor Alice has recommended. Donald Alexander is an internist who specializes in HIV/AIDS. I like the way the receptionist sounds when I call and make an appointment for Monday, April 3. The beats of my heart slow back down to a steady rhythm.

On that Monday, I remind Dennis that I will come home from work at lunchtime so that we can go to the doctor at 1:00. With kisses goodbye, I leave the house at 7:00 while everyone else is just getting up for school.

It's 8:45 and things have finally calmed down in the office. Mail bag in hand, I am filling teachers' mail boxes with the day's delivery when I hear the phone ring.

"Good morning, Thomas Jefferson High School. How may I help you?"

"Scott, Samuel's throwing up blood, and I don't know what to do."

"Dennis, what do you mean, throwing up blood? Where is he?"

"He's in the shower. In fact, he's crumbled in the corner, crying. Says his stomach hurts."

Overhearing me, Mary is quickly at my desk. "Joan, go home. Whatever it is, just go. We'll take care of everything here."

"Dennis, can you get him to the hospital, to the ER? I can meet you there."

"I don't think I have the energy to get there; I'm already exhausted. I'll help him get out of the shower and then William will take him to the ER. Presbyterian?"

"Okay. Yes, Presbyterian. I'm leaving now. Will you be able to get him out of the shower?"

"William will help me. Isn't today my doctor's appointment? What are you going to do about that?"

"Yes, your appointment is at 1:00 so I don't know. Let's see what they say about Samuel first; I'll call you from the hospital."

Heart pounding, I run to the car. Outside the ER, William pulls up with Samuel just as I'm opening my door. We each put a hand under a shoulder and shepherd Samuel into the ER.

After checking Samuel in with the nurse, I phone my new insurance company to make the necessary contact for a patient being seen in the emergency room. As I explain that my enrollment date was just two days ago, Saturday, April 1, my heart begins to beat faster. Once I am assured that everything is in order, I return to Samuel who has been ushered into a treatment room. A young doctor comes into the room. "Mrs. Curtis, I am Dr. Stewart. What seems to be the problem with Samuel?"

"Samuel, honey, will you tell Dr. Stewart when all this started? I was at work when my husband called and said Samuel was in the shower, doubled over in pain and throwing up blood."

Dr. Stewart conducts an examination and asks me to go out into the hall to talk. "He is obviously quite tender, but I don't feel anything that I can pinpoint. I'm going to send him down for a CT scan because I'm thinking maybe appendicitis. If that is confirmed, we'll have to operate to remove the appendix."

"Dr. Stewart, my husband is sick; he has AIDS and his first doctor's appointment with his new doctor is this afternoon at 1:00. I cannot leave Samuel, but Dennis cannot miss this doctor's appointment either. How long do you think it will take for the CT scan so that you'll know what you have to do?" Feeling the tears form, I close my eyes for a minute. *God, keep me strong. I'm doing all I can, and I need you to fill me with strength.*

"We'll get Samuel down right away for the scan, Mrs. Curtis." He puts his hands on my shoulders and looks right into my eyes. "We'll move as quickly as we can; I promise. Now, let's go back in and explain everything to Samuel."

At 10:00, Samuel is taken down for the CT scan. Nothing definitive can be seen so Dr. Stewart decides to wait it out for a little while explaining that they don't want to operate un-necessarily, but they don't want to dismiss him when he is obviously in pain. By now it is 11:15, and I don't feel like I can leave Samuel when nothing has been decided. I call our friends Rob and Annie Long who agree to pick up Dennis and take him to the doctor where I'll meet him. That way, I can stay at the hospital for another hour or so.

At 12:40 we are still in a holding pattern, and I know I have to leave. Samuel understands that

I have to leave. Dr. Stewart and another physician who has joined us, Dr. Roberts, also understand that I have to leave. I'm looking at my sixteen-year-old son lying on a bed in the emergency room, and I don't understand why I have to leave him there. I don't understand why all this is happening. Drs. Stewart and Roberts walk me out of the ER, each assuring me that they will take care of Samuel. I can't stop the tears now, and Dr. Stewart hugs me. "We won't let anything happen to him. You go take care of your husband."

I meet Dennis at the office of Dr. Donald Alexander. After just fifteen minutes with him, I know he is everything you want in a doctor when you are dealing with a terminal illness. He is kind, compassionate, and thorough. Balancing five children and their activities can be overwhelming under the best of circumstances, and these circumstances are anything but ideal. Fortunately, I have been devoted to keeping a medical journal of rashes, ulcers, fevers, weight loss, fatigue—everything Dennis has been battling these last few months. I also have made notes of medications, hospitalizations—really anything and everything related to Dennis. I knew I couldn't remember it all. Dr. Alexander gets a good history from me, conducts a thorough examination, and diagnoses Dennis with Mycobacterium tuberculosis—a type of tuberculosis associated with HIV/AIDS. It both destroys red blood cells and affects absorption of nutrients, which results in severe weight loss. He prescribes a new medication, schedules a transfusion of red blood cells, and requests another appointment in two weeks.

Dennis is exhausted when we leave, but he needs to see Samuel so we head back to the hospital after calling William to pick up Drew and Elizabeth from school and get them something for dinner. We get back to the hospital about 3:30, and they've decided to do the appendectomy. Dr. Stewart explains that he is still not one hundred percent sure of the diagnosis, but they are close enough that the surgery is on. Samuel is wheeled to surgery about 4:30 and is in his room by 6:30. Dennis is absolutely exhausted, but I know he had to be here for Samuel. He crawls onto the bed with Samuel, and they doze off together, side by side.

Suddenly, I remember that the Dallas Cup is in one week, and Samuel was going to get to play for the first time. Dallas Cup is the largest international youth soccer tournament in the world, and Samuel was so excited; it was the one good thing happening in his life. We have even committed to hosting two players from Argentina for the week. So now what? Samuel cannot play; Dennis has an appointment for a blood transfusion next week; we'll have two additional young men in the house. I look at Dennis and Samuel sleeping. Every ounce of energy is gone. Is there room for three in that bed? I wake Dennis up, kiss Samuel good-bye, and we leave. *Please, God, watch over Samuel tonight, and give me strength for whatever comes tomorrow.*

Samuel is released on Wednesday; he doesn't mind missing the week of school but is visibly upset that he will not be able to play in the Cup. Dennis and I assure him that one of us will make sure he gets to the games his team plays and that the players from Argentina can still stay with us. We are sticking to our commitment of keeping things as normal as possible for the kids. Dennis is sicker, but that has become part of the normal. The boys, Alejandro and Javier, arrive on Sunday; Javier speaks English; Alejandro doesn't. I can see a change in Samuel once they arrive. His face is relaxed, and that twinkle is back in his eyes. Drew, too, is excited that they are here and in our house. They are handsome and engaging young men, and my heart is happy that we went ahead with this plan.

CHAPTER 10

The Cure-all—A Puppy

The days pass quickly as I am busy with work and managing things at home. Because we left the washer and dryer in Virginia, I am washing clothes for six at the laundromat. I really want to be back in our house so I again contact the people who have rented it, and they agree to move out at the end of June. Mary needs a clerk each morning for the summer, and I agree to work since that means additional income. I receive my first paycheck on April 15. Because insurance premiums for two months were deducted, my paycheck amounts to $10.86. I have to laugh; what else is there to do. Dennis can't believe it and wants to frame it. I explain that we are out of milk and bread; I need the $10.86.

I can't complain. Dennis has received three transfusions of red blood cells and does have more energy. He is eating a little better but still seems to be losing weight. Dr. Alexander sees him every two weeks and, in addition to the medication, he decides to use steroids in an attempt to build muscle and add weight. The medicine Dennis is on requires weekly monitoring of liver function so a nurse comes every Tuesday to draw blood. We have not had to pay anything for his care.

We do receive notice at the end of May that the insurance will not pay for Samuel's surgery and hospitalization because he was admitted through the emergency room and required notification was not made. I immediately send a letter in response, recounting the events of April 3, which include my phone call to the insurance company before Samuel is admitted. Within two weeks, I receive another notice that they will pay for the first night but not the second night. I write a second letter stating that my son is sixteen years old and his surgery was at 4:30 in the afternoon. I ask the question: who is going to watch him the next day at home since his father is dying and his mother is working to support the family. I don't hear any more from the insurance company, and I receive no bills from the hospital or doctors. Certainly, life could be easier, but I cannot complain because we have insurance.

Kathryn comes home in mid-May and is horrified by the change in her father. Because she's been in Switzerland this past semester, I have kept letters light and newsy. She didn't need to have this time ruined by worry. She's not happy with me because she's always been a child who just wanted to know the truth, but she seems to understand my reasoning, and we move on. She gets a job waiting tables at The Olive Garden and spends many evenings with Scott, her boyfriend of four years.

Right before Mother's Day, Dennis and William come home with a surprise for everyone—

a puppy! She is darling, her name is Sam, and I am absolutely furious. What is he thinking or is he even thinking? That virus must have invaded his brain! He breaks Elizabeth's heart by making us leave Shiski in Virginia and now he gets a puppy—one we have to house train! My gosh! We're in a rented house; I'm working at TJ full-time; I have to go the laundromat to wash clothes; I'm responsible for five children, two of whom are so at odds with each other you can feel it in the air; and he brings home a puppy for me to take care of! You've got to be kidding!

Drew and Elizabeth are thrilled, but I can't think of a civil thing to say. "Isn't she cute? I named her Sam after your dad. I just thought we needed a little happiness for Mother's Day." He is pleading with me, but I am too mad. I don't even care that Elizabeth and Drew are in love with this puppy, and Samuel and Kathryn are not far behind them. I just can't take care of one more thing. I walk out of the den and go lie down in our bedroom. Everyone else stays in the den to oooh and ahhh over our new family member, Sam.

I must doze off because I am suddenly awakened with the sound of a puppy peeing. Bounding from the bed, I see Sam just as she finishes messing up the carpet. Seething, I pound into the den where I find Dennis lying on the sofa, eyes closed, and Kathryn curled up in the chair reading. Arms crossed, I look straight at Dennis. "Your dog just peed on the carpet in the bedroom. You better get up and clean it before it soaks in and smells." I turn and walk out the front door, letting it slam behind me.

I hear Dennis say to Kathryn, "I think I've really pissed her off this time."

It takes me about two days to let my guard down, but once I do, I, too, fall in love with Sam. When Elizabeth puts a leash around her to walk her, she just sits her little bottom on the ground, resulting in being dragged. The rest of us, watching, can't stop laughing. Black and white with cute little perky ears and the brightest eyes, I love that she has the same name as my father. Honestly, Dennis Curtis has always known just what to say and do to get me. What is my life going to be like when he's not here to do these kinds of things?

Once school is out; there is increasing tension between William and Samuel. I request that William move into an apartment, and he finds something small, which he can afford on the salary he's earning as a bartender. Samuel, Drew, and Elizabeth are glad to be out of school, and life settles into a routine. Dennis and I just have one car between us so he takes me to work and picks me up at 12:00. It will really help when Samuel can drive again.

One afternoon when Dennis picks me up, I can tell he's been somewhere before getting me. "Where did you go this morning?"

"How do you know I've been anywhere?"

"I don't know how, but I can tell. What's up?"

"Well, I had an appointment with the IRS this morning."

"The IRS? Why?"

"Well, I didn't pay our personal taxes in 1988 because I chose to take care of the payroll taxes instead. I went in to let them know I couldn't do anything about it now."

"What did they say? What did you say?"

"I told them I had AIDS and would probably be dead by September. They said they were sorry."

"So can they do anything? What can happen?"

"They're not going to do anything, Joan. It's been seven years, and now they know I'm dying. You're not going to hear from them." I'm not sure if I do believe him, but it seems I don't have much choice.

Because we know we'll be back in our own house by fall, Samuel rides with Dennis one day to get an athletic physical done at TJ; he wants to play soccer in the fall. When the nurse Tommie Allen goes through the litany of usual questions and asks about thoughts of suicide, Samuel answers truthfully; yes, he's thought about killing himself. Tommie finishes the physical and then comes across to the front office to talk to me about taking Samuel to a psychologist for an evaluation. "I cannot release him to play soccer until I have a psych evaluation in my hand."

I call the insurance company, and they agree to four mental health visits initially. I get the name of an adolescent psychiatrist because Samuel and I have been down this road before, and if medication is prescribed, I just want to deal with one doctor. We have enough doctor visits with Dennis. After an extensive evaluation, Samuel is diagnosed with bipolar depression and put on lithium. His psychiatrist explains the dangers of lithium to both Samuel and me; an overdose will kill you. For the time being, I decide to keep the medication and give it to Samuel one dose at a time. I don't even take time to think about what "bipolar depression" entails or what all of the ramifications might be. We have a diagnosis; we have a medication; that's all I can take in right now.

CHAPTER 11

A Downward Spiral

One day in mid-June, Dennis and Elizabeth pick me up, and Dennis doesn't look right. "Are you okay?"

"I don't know. I … uh, I can't seem to keep my thoughts straight, I … I … something's not right … not right." He gets out of the car.

I head over to the driver's side. "Let me drive. We're going to see Donald right now. Get in the car, Dennis, so we can get there before they leave for lunch." Dennis gets in but is still agitated and mumbling.

"What's wrong with Daddy, Mommy? What's wrong?" Elizabeth, in the back seat, starts crying.

"I don't know, Honey, but it'll be okay; we're taking him to the doctor right now. It's okay,

Sweet Pea." I can't drive fast enough because I am really scared. We pull into the parking lot just as Donald pulls out of the lot and his nurse, John, is getting in his car. By this time, Elizabeth is hysterical, and I'm not far behind her. John takes one look at us and comes right over.

"I'll take Dennis in and call Donald. Is there someone at home to take care of Elizabeth so you can take her home? I'll stay with Dennis until Donald gets here; he'll be okay."

Samuel is at home so I leave Dennis with John and take Elizabeth home to Samuel. I don't have time to explain. "Dad's having some kind of attack so he's at Dr. Alexander's office, and I had to get Elizabeth out of there because she doesn't need to see all that. Dad's okay; they just need to figure out what's happening. I'll call you." I hug them both, reminding them that I love them, and race back to Donald's office.

By the time I get back, Donald has returned and determined that Dennis has gone into a steroid mania. Donald has given Dennis an injection of Halidol to stop the mania and to make him sleep, which Dennis is already doing. Donald tells me, "Stop the steroids; he can't take them."

I remind Donald, "I know Dennis is losing ground, and I do want to know the truth. When it's time to stop all medication, don't pacify me; just tell me, okay? I can take anything you tell me."

"Don't give up yet, Joan. There are still some things to try. I'll tell you when it's time. I promise."

John and Donald help me get Dennis to the car, and we put him in lying down in the back seat. Once I get home, Samuel helps me get him to the bed. I don't bother taking his clothes off; I just pull down the covers; Samuel gets him situated in the bed; I pull up the covers. Then Elizabeth and I curl up together on the other side so we don't disturb him but are next to him. We lie still for about thirty minutes, and Elizabeth drifts off to sleep. I gently get out of bed and go talk to Samuel and Drew.

Just after dinner, the phone rings. "Joan, this is John, Donald's nurse."

"Hi, John. Dennis is okay; in fact, he's still asleep."

"That's good, Joan, but I didn't call to check on Dennis. I called to check on you. I don't know how you're doing this. When I saw your little one today, I just thought … I don't know. I want to know how you're doing. You're the one we have to take care of."

"I'm okay, John. I'm taking one day at a time and some days, like today, I take an hour at a time. Right now I can't stop and think; I just have to keep moving."

"I know. We care about you, Joan; don't forget that. Sleep well, and give us a call if you need anything. Donald and I, we're both here."

"Thank you, John. Thank you for taking care of Dennis today so I could get Elizabeth out of there. Good night." Hanging up the phone, I know I will never forget this phone call to check on me.

Dennis sleeps through the night and doesn't wake up until the next afternoon. When he does wake up, he remembers nothing of the day before.

A few days later, it is the Saturday before Father's Day. Dennis decides he wants to go to Longview to see my mother. I ask him about the kids—his kids—but he insists he wants just the two of us to go. "I want to see your mother, go to the cemetery and talk to your dad, and eat at Johnny Cace's. Father's Day means I can do what I want to do, and that is what I want to do." I call Mother, give Kathryn thirty dollars to take everyone to a movie and to Ball's Hamburgers, and we are set to go. We drive down early, visit with Mother and take a casual walk around the yard where I grew up. Dennis pauses at the gate by Daddy's garden and runs his hand gently over the sign I put there in 1968, "Sam's

Paradise." Mother and I stand at the back sliding glass door and watch; it's as if he's imprinting everything on his memory one last time. Following a brief nap for Dennis, we eat a mid-afternoon dinner at Cace's. Dennis has always loved oysters but has not eaten them for fifteen months; oysters can carry bacteria that are deadly to anyone with a suppressed immune system. He points to "Oysters on the half-shell" on the menu and looks at me with eyebrows raised.

"What the heck! Go for it," I answer.

Grabbing my hand, Dennis replies, "I'm so lucky that you love me."

"Yes, you are." I order a martini for him and think of all the martini nights that he has shared with my mother and father. They couldn't have loved Dennis more if he had been their own son. And my father was the father Dennis always wanted but had to wait until he married me to get. After dinner, we go to the cemetery, take Mother home and head back to Dallas. Dennis sleeps the whole way, and I'm grateful that we've had such a good day.

Two days later, Dennis is not feeling well at all. He doesn't get out of bed and by 5:30 is calling me to come back to the bedroom. "I don't think I can breathe. I need to go to the hospital." He is clammy and is short of breath. His eyes reveal fear.

I know Donald's out of the office by now so I call a friend from our neighborhood who is a nurse. Lynne comes over and takes a quick look. "His breathing is a little shallow and his blood pressure's low. Go ahead and call an ambulance so you don't have to wait around forever in the ER, but you have time and don't need to panic. Do you want me to stay?"

"No, I'm okay. Thank you so much, Lynne. I didn't know what to do." I walk her to the door. I go back to Dennis and pick up the phone to call for an ambulance.

"Border's Books. How may I help you?"

"What number is this?" The voice on the phone gives out numbers that don't match at all what I've dialed. "I'm sorry; I must have misdialed." I hang up and dial again, carefully.

"Border's Books. How may I help you?"

By now I am starting to panic. "I'm trying to call 214-385-7483, but I keep getting you. What's wrong with the phone?"

"I'm sorry, Ma'am, but the line must be scrambling the numbers. Why don't you wait a few minutes and try again."

Dennis' breathing is shallower or maybe it's my imagination. I don't know, but I am scared. I wait a few minutes and dial the number again. "Border's Books. How may I help you?"

I don't even say anything; I just hang up and dial zero.

"I'm trying to call an ambulance for my husband but keep getting another number and I know I'm dialing the right number but I guess the line is scrambling the numbers and I don't know what to do but I need an ambulance now. I ..."

"Yes, Ma'am, I'll call an ambulance for you. What address is that?" the operator is speaking so gently that I begin to calm down automatically.

"4538 Thunder Road in Dallas. We need to go to Baylor Hospital."

"Yes, Ma'am. I'll get that ambulance right now. Don't worry; I'm taking care of it."

I hang up and quickly pack a few things for Dennis. Then I go tell the kids what's going on and sit down to wait. Within fifteen minutes the ambulance is there, and Dennis is loaded into it and is on his way to Baylor in another five minutes. Promising the kids that I'll call soon and blowing them kisses, I follow the ambulance in my car.

Upon arrival at Baylor, Dennis is checked in; Donald is called and there within thirty minutes; Dennis is assessed, admitted, and sent to a room. It has all happened so fast my head is spinning. Donald assures me that this is not the end. "He's just not getting enough nourishment and he's dehydrated. We'll get some fluids and nutrients into him by IV, and you can take him home in four or five days. Don't give up yet; it's not time."

Because we are both exhausted and he has a roommate this time, I don't stay too long. I also know the kids are anxious. Once I make sure he's resting comfortably, I head home so I can update everyone and try to get some sleep. Tomorrow I'll bring the kids so they can see that their dad is okay.

The first thing the next morning, I go to TJ and tell Mary that I am not going to be able to work this week because I need to be at the hospital with Dennis. I call Dennis to check on him and, hearing that he is feeling better, tell him that I will take care of some things at home this morning and then bring Drew and Elizabeth by after lunch.

By the time I finish all the loose ends at home and fix some lunch for the kids, it is 2:00 before we head downtown to Baylor. Elizabeth is so excited about seeing her daddy that she is jabbering all the way to his room. The door is closed, and I caution Elizabeth to open it slowly and caution Drew to keep his voice lowered because Daddy does have a roommate this time. As soon as we walk in, I know it is not good. The roommate appears to be asleep so we tiptoe to Dennis' side of the curtain. Lying on his back, he is unnaturally white, and, although his eyes are closed, I can tell from one quick glance that he is feeling lethargic. "Dennis, Drew and Elizabeth are here." I walk over and kiss him on the cheek.

"I don't feel right, Scott. I felt okay when I woke up this morning but now, I don't know; I don't feel good, like something's wrong, and I need more than oxygen." He doesn't say anything to the kids, which lets me know he is really in bad shape.

Elizabeth comes to where I am standing by the bed and hides behind me. "Mommy, I want to go home now."

"Don't you want to say hello to Daddy?" I try to coax her from behind me, but she won't budge.

"I just want to go, Mommy. Please, can we go home now?" Elizabeth starts to cry, and I know I have to get her out of here because she is frightened. Drew has walked over to Dennis' bed and is holding his hand.

"Hey, guys, let's get out of here and let Daddy rest. I don't think he slept well last night so maybe it's better if we go home and let him sleep. We can come back tomorrow." I take both Drew and Elizabeth into the hall, "You all stand right here while I go in and make sure Daddy is comfortable and tell him I'll be back in a little while." I am actually a little uneasy leaving Dennis so I use the phone at the nurses' station and call home. "Samuel, do you think you can come get Drew and Elizabeth? I don't want to leave Dad, and this is too frightening for Elizabeth." Samuel doesn't have a car, but Kathryn is home and she says she'll come and get them. She doesn't have to be at work until 4:00 so there is time. We take the elevator downstairs to the lobby and wait for Kathryn.

I make sure both Drew and Elizabeth are calm and that Samuel will be home to stay with them when Kathryn goes to work. I give her some money to get hamburgers for dinner. I watch Kathryn drive away and then head back into the hospital and back up to Dennis' room.

By the time I get upstairs, Donald is coming out of the room. Footsteps clicking down the hall, I pick up my pace so Donald does not get away before I can talk to him. "Donald, what do you think about Dennis? He doesn't seem to be doing very well."

"Hi, Joan. Dennis is holding his own right now. The oxygen has made breathing a little easier for him, although the Mycobacterium is really taking its toll. He will have an infusion of red blood cells tomorrow, but I do see a new problem now, Joan. The virus has gone into his brain, I believe. I can't be sure yet, but I do see definite signs. This will require more of you, Joan, in terms of patience and being the primary decision-maker. I'm going to write orders for the red cell infusion, and I'll be back later tonight before I go home. Do you have any questions?"

"Is it time, Donald? Is it time to say stop the meds?"

"No, Joan, not yet. I will tell you when it's time. I promise." Donald heads to the nurses' station, and I go in and sit with Dennis. As I watch him sleep, I realize that I need a friend. I quietly leave the room and find a phone to call Alice. Without hesitation, she volunteers to drive down and have dinner with me. I then call home to check in with the kids.

"Drew, it's Momma. How is everything there?"

"It's okay, Momma. Kathryn gave us money to get hamburgers. Is that okay?"

"Yes, Honey, that's fine. Is Elizabeth there, Drew? What's she doing?"

"Samuel's been playing Uno with her, but now she's just watching TV. That's what we're all doing, Momma. Samuel put a movie on for us, and William's gonna take us to get burgers when he gets off work. Suma called about the Comet tryouts, but I wrote it all down. When are you coming home?"

"I'll be home about 8:00, Honey. Alice is going to come see Daddy and then we're going to get dinner. I'll make sure Daddy is resting comfortably before I come home. Let me talk to Samuel, please." I give the same information to Samuel and then talk quickly to Elizabeth so I can assure her that Daddy is feeling okay and assure myself that she is feeling okay.

When I get back to Dennis' room, Blair Monie is there. Blair is the senior pastor at our church, Preston Hollow Presbyterian, and since I hear Blair and Dennis talking, I remain quietly outside the room. After a few minutes, I walk in, greet Blair, and thank him for coming. He asks Dennis if a prayer would be okay, and when Dennis nods okay, the three of us take each other's hands and bow our heads. I then walk Blair to the elevator, and when I tell him that I will leave shortly, he insists on waiting for me so he can walk me to my car. Eyes only half-open, I can tell Dennis is really tired so I kiss him goodnight. "Sleep well, my love. I'll come back in the morning but will leave the kids at home. I think the hospital scares Elizabeth."

"You're right, and I don't think Drew needs to be here, either. In fact, I don't want any of the kids to come here, but I need you, Scott, so do come early, please. Are you parked close to the hospital?"

"Blair is waiting for me; he's going to walk me to my car. I'll see you tomorrow." Leaning down to kiss him again, I whisper, "I love you, Dennis. Let that be your last thought tonight."

The next morning I get to the hospital by 9:00, and Dennis' roommate is not in his bed. Eyes open wide, Dennis is visibly shaken when

I move the curtain. "Honey, what happened? Where's your roommate?"

"Dead. He had a heart attack last night. It was horrible. They brought that crash cart and kept working on him, but he was gone and then they left him in the room the rest of the night. I asked the nurse to move him, but she said they were waiting for his family to get here before they moved him. Scott, it was so violent. I don't want to die like that, okay? Don't let me die like that."

I take him in my arms and hold him tightly. Feeling the shaking of his body, I kiss his face lightly and continue holding him tightly. I want to squeeze the fear out of him, but I don't know how. *God, help me now. Please help me now. Help me be strong and unafraid so Dennis can take strength from me. I know You will not let me fall, so help me give something to Dennis.*

Kathryn does not go into work until late afternoon, so I can spend the day with Dennis. We are quiet; he takes frequent naps, and I read, keeping the chair right by his bed so I can reach out and touch him if I need to reassure him. Samuel calls late in the afternoon and tells me he will order pizza and watch a movie with Drew and Elizabeth so I can stay at the hospital. *Thank You, God, for blessing me with these amazing children. I can be strong because not only do You give me strength, my children give me strength.*

I know I need to get out of the hospital for a little while, and I need someone to discuss the day with so I can sleep tonight. There are only two people who can help me right now, Alice and Becky. I know Becky's daughter is getting married on Saturday, but I call anyway. I've taken so much of Alice's time already.

Becky doesn't hesitate. She comes right down, and we go to dinner. Two hours of nonstop talking mixed with tears, and I am exhausted. Becky goes home, and I go back up to Dennis' room, tired but renewed. Thank you, Becky.

Saturday morning I am at the hospital when Donald stops to see Dennis. "I think the infusion of red blood cells has done its work on the anemia. Dennis, you've got to eat more, and, Joan, just get him to eat whatever he will eat. I think one more day with us, and if everything looks good in the morning, you can go home." Now this is good news!

Alice comes down late morning and visits with Dennis and then we go get lunch. "Joan, are you going to Alyson's wedding tonight? Do you need help with the kids?" Becky's daughter is getting married, but I don't want to leave Dennis alone; nights scare him.

"I don't think I can go. Kathryn has to work, but Samuel will be home with Drew and Elizabeth. I just worry about Dennis in the evening if he's left alone to worry about what's ahead. If I stay until he's ready to sleep, then we can talk through those fears before they are out of control."

"Joan, I'll come back and sit with Dennis. You need to be at Alyson's wedding. She is Becky's daughter, and you need to be there. For you and for Becky. Think of the history of your friendship with Becky and Dave. After their son committed suicide, you were there every day with Becky, making sure she ate, listening to Doug's service on tape, doing whatever you could to make sure she wasn't alone. You and Elizabeth spent the whole first year of Elizabeth's life with Becky. You cannot miss her daughter's wedding. Besides, a wedding will be a good change of scenery for you. What if I come back at 5:00? Is that early enough?"

With that plan in place, I spend the afternoon with Dennis and leave about 4:30 so I can shower and get dressed for the wedding. Everything is beautiful, and I catch Becky's eye as she is escorted down the aisle. A simple nod of the head says it all. I am sitting by myself, and I make myself stay focused on the moment. "In sickness and in health." The words wash over me as I hear them. Dennis and I will celebrate our twenty-third wedding anniversary in a few weeks. It's hard to remember when we weren't married, but in another way, it seems like just yesterday that it was me standing up there promising to love him "for richer and poorer, in sickness and in health, for as long as you both shall live."

I go to the reception just long enough to speak to Alyson and Tim, the bride and groom, and my dear friends, Becky and Dave. Standing on my tiptoes, I put my arms around Dave's neck. "Thank you for sharing Becky with me the other night. I know this was not the week to ask her to come to the hospital."

Gently removing my arms from his neck, Dave holds me so that he is holding my gaze in his. "Joan, when Doug died seven years ago, you were the one constant for Becky. If you had not stayed beside her, I don't know if we would even have Becky to share with you. Maybe in some small way, we've been able to give back to you what you gave to us then." That is it for me.

Quickly hugging Becky again, I am back in the car and headed to the hospital to hold Dennis until he falls asleep.

Dennis is discharged Sunday morning, and all the kids are there to welcome him home. He does look better, rested with some color back in his face. The relief is evident on the faces of the older kids when they really look at him. We all sit in the den for awhile, laughing with Elizabeth as she tries to teach puppy Sam some tricks. I have to admit, as mad as I was about that puppy when Dennis brought her home, she is certainly a breath of fresh air for us right now.

After lunch, Dennis lies down and quickly falls asleep. I sit on the side of the bed watching him. I don't know how much longer we have, but I do know I don't want him back in the hospital. He is so much more comfortable here at home. I also know that this involves the kids, too, and maybe it's too much for them to have him this sick at home. My head is spinning. Do

I just make this decision for everyone? Should I ask them what they want? If they tell me it's too much to have him at home, will I really do something different or will I just ignore what they've said? What do I do? What do I do? *I'm at a loss here, God. Where is the instruction book? What if the older kids say one thing and the younger kids say another? Help me, God. Help me.*"

Drew is ready for his second day of try-outs for the Comets soccer team. The Comets are a long-standing first class competitive soccer organization, and Drew really wants a spot on this team. His best friend Bradley Napper plays for the Comets, and Drew not only wants to play on a team with Bradley, he wants his own skill recognized by earning a Comets' position. Being called back for this second tryout has offered him more than a glimmer of hope; he has an air of confidence as he jumps in the car.

The try-out goes well, and we go home to wait for the phone call. I can't imagine that he won't make the team. He is a skilled player, and the coach, David Hudgel knows how hard Drew works because David has seen him at the Napper house and watched the boys practice. Few of the boys at this age have a kick as strong as Drew's, and anybody can see he has a head for the game. Drew anticipates where the ball is going next. I've never understood how he does that, but he does. Something good is going to happen, and we are all ready for something good.

The following afternoon, I answer the phone and immediately hear the apologetic tone in the coach's voice. "Drew is a really good player, one of the best, but we just don't need another defensive player this year."

My heart is breaking, but I've got to say something. "Would Drew have to play defense? He can play forward."

"Drew is a natural defender. I could put him on the team, but he wouldn't get much playing time, and Drew needs to play. You get better by playing, not by sitting on the bench. I'm sorry. I really would love to have him and work with him, but it just doesn't make sense for this year."

"Okay, I do understand." But I don't understand. This is the perfect year that it makes sense. Drew's father is dying; put him on the team just to give him another place to focus. But I don't say that. "Thank you for calling." I hang up the phone and walk down the hall to Drew's room. What in the world am I going to tell him?

"Honey, David called. They don't need another defender this year, so it's not going to work out with the Comets." His shoulders drop and the sadness in his face is too much to bear. "I know you're disappointed. I am so sorry." I don't see any disappointment, only sadness. "We'll find another team. I'll call Suma, and she'll tell me teams that are looking for players. And not just any team, but a good team. Some team is going to be lucky to get you."

He walks over to me, and I take him in my arms just as the tears start to fall. I hold him as his whole body rocks with deep sobs. We walk over to the bed and sit. We cry together until we are both out of tears.

Later that night, I find Kathryn sitting on her bed, crying. She had been out with Scott, the young man she's been dating for four years, and I'm surprised to find her at home. Sitting down beside her, I ask, "Honey, what's wrong? Where's Scott?"

"I broke up with him, Mom." Her tears are coming faster.

"What happened? Do you want to talk?" I pull her close to me.

"I don't know, Mom. It just seems we don't have anything in common anymore. We don't have anything to say to each other. That's what I told Scott. That it seems like he'd always rather be somewhere else. How can all the years we've been together just evaporate like that? I don't get it. I just know I hurt. I hurt so much."

I don't know what to say to her because I know nothing I say will ease the hurt right now. That much I understand, so I do what my mother did all those years ago when my heart was broken. I take her in my arms and hold her until she has cried herself to sleep.

It seems that having Dennis near the end of his life is not enough to keep the world at bay. No, the world just keeps turning, and all the hurts that maybe won't matter much in thirty years, hurt deeply right now.

CHAPTER 12

The Beginning of the End

Dennis has not eaten much since coming home from the hospital because he just doesn't have any energy and even eating seems to be too much for him. Wednesday morning I call Donald, and he prescribes a new medicine to combat the fatigue by fortifying the red blood cells. Dennis wants to get out of the house, so he rides with me to the drug store. We decide to stop by Tom Thumb, the grocery store, before we go home. "I can't go in, Scott, my hair is dirty."

Dennis' clothes are falling off of his one hundred and fifteen pound body, and he's worried about his hair being dirty? The absurdity of it all makes me laugh. I reach into the back seat and grab Samuel's cap. "Here, Honey, wear this. It'll hide your dirty hair." When we get into the store, I see Ray Stanley, a teacher's aide at Thomas Jefferson.

"Hi, Ray. This is my husband, Dennis. Dennis, Ray Stanley."

"Hello, Ray," Dennis puts his hand out to shake Ray's hand. "I hope you're having a good summer."

Grasping Dennis' hand, she responds, "Yes, I am, Dennis. It's nice to meet you. How are you feeling these days?" Ray Stanley is the teacher's aide in the classroom where our neighbor made the comment about Dennis having AIDS and people should stay away from him. This act of kindness she displays when she takes his hand helps me see that she is a person of compassion. She doesn't run in the other direction, and she is not afraid to touch him. This brief interchange helps me to know that I want to know her.

"Oh, I'm holding on most days. I'm feeling good enough for grocery shopping."

"Well, then, you must be in fine shape. No one goes to the grocery if you can get out of it."

"Yes, so we better get what we came for," I chime in to the conversation. "It's good to see you, Ray. Enjoy the rest of your summer."

"You, too, Curtis family. I'll see you in August, Joan."

We quickly get the few things we need and head home. Dennis takes his medicine, and being completely exhausted by the running around, lies down on the couch in the den. "Don't you want to go get in the bed, Honey?"

"No, I want to lie right here. I've been gone too much, and I want to lie right here in the middle of everyone and everything."

With his head in my lap, he naps while the rest of us watch a movie. Elizabeth sits on the other side of me and gently pats her daddy's head every once in a while.

To the delight of everybody, I make manicotti for dinner. Dennis even eats a little and keeps it all down. Elizabeth really wants to watch one of her Disney movies, so after dinner we put another movie on and laugh through *Escape to Witch Mountain*. It isn't a funny movie, but Samuel, Kathryn, Dennis, and I keep making comments about scenes that evoke memories of past viewings. This was the first videotape that we bought, and that was in 1983. After the movie I tuck the younger kids in, and Dennis is ready for bed, too. I get in bed with Dennis before he falls asleep, and it is good to feel his arms around me. He falls asleep rather quickly, and I lie next to him for a while. It's been a good day. A really good day. *Thank You, God.*

Thursday is uneventful except that Dennis is feeling nauseated again, so he doesn't want to eat anything or take the medicine. By mid-afternoon, he finally concedes to eat a little toast so he'll have something in his stomach and can take the medicine. Within fifteen minutes, he has lost both the medicine and the toast. "That's it, Scott, I can't do this. That medicine is no good if I can't even keep it down, and, frankly, I'll take tired over nausea any day."

There is no reason to argue because he's the one who has to live with it, and because I do understand what he's saying about the fruitlessness of taking medicine to throw it back up again. I'll take most minor aches and pains over nausea. Calling Donald can wait until morning. I don't want to go anywhere for a new prescription today, and I've got other thoughts rolling around in my head.

On Friday, July 7, the thought that has been buried deep within my brain comes to the forefront—is Dennis going to live long enough for Kathryn to go back to school in Ohio and still have time with him when she comes home? It is an important question because I do not want her to lose any more time with him, but it is her senior year, and I don't want her to stop now and fail to go back and finish. This is something

I want to ask Donald about because I need more information to make an intelligent decision. Since I need to let Donald know that Dennis is not taking the most recently prescribed medicine because it nauseated him, I decide this is the perfect time to call and ask about Kathryn's situation. Picking up the telephone, I dial the number for Donald's office.

"Hi, John,, this is Joan Curtis. Is Donald available to talk for a minute?" John puts me on hold, and in just a couple of minutes, Donald picks up the phone.

"Hi, Joan. What's going on with Dennis?"

"Donald, that last medicine you prescribed nauseated Dennis so he hasn't taken any since Wednesday morning. He also cannot keep any food down so he's basically given up trying to eat. I'm worried about his weight because even I can see that it is way too low, and he's got to have some nourishment. Honestly, I had to help him out of the shower this morning because he doesn't have any strength, and he looks like he's from one of the videos of the liberation of a concentration camp. Is there anything that can help him keep some food down and increase his appetite, too?"

"I'll call in something for him, Joan, but you have to know that this is about the last thing we can try. You've got to make sure he takes the full dose for it to do any good, okay?"

"Thank you, Donald. And there's one other thing I need to ask you about; I need some advice before I say anything. Our older daughter, Kathryn, is in college in Ohio, and she'll begin her senior year this fall. I'm not sure what to tell her to do. If Dennis is going to live for at least another year or two, then I want her to go back to school and finish. But if you think he's going to die within the next several months, then maybe I should ask her to stay home and postpone her senior year for a while."

"Joan, Dennis is going to be gone before she leaves for school."

"No, Donald, you didn't understand; Kathryn leaves for school in six weeks."

"Joan, Dennis is going to be gone before she leaves for school because he'll be gone within the next month. You've always asked me to be honest with you, Joan, and I am being honest and forthright. Dennis probably doesn't have more than a month left."

I can't seem to catch my breath, but somehow I manage to talk, "Thank you, Donald. Thank you for your honesty. If you will go ahead and call in that medicine, I'll go pick it up right now."

"I'll ask John to call it in as soon as I hang up, and I'll check back with you Monday morning. I'm just going to write the script for four days of medication, and then if it does some good, I'll give you more on Monday, okay? And, Joan, I'm going to ask them to deliver the prescription, and I want you to get some rest this weekend."

My head is spinning as I hang up the phone. *A month? A month? Dennis will be dead in a month?* I pick up the phone and call my sister in Houston. "Judy, I need you to come to Dallas this weekend. Can you come?"

"What's wrong, Joan? Is Dennis okay? Of course, I can come."

"I just talked to Donald, Dennis' doctor, and he told me Dennis only had a month left. I need you, Judy. I really need you with me."

"I'm coming. Just give me a few minutes to make sure everything is taken care of here, and then I'm on the next flight. You don't need to pick me up; I'll just rent a car."

Now the tears are on the verge, but I hold them back. I can't fall apart now. "Thank you, Judy. I'll see you in a little while."

"Hang on, Joan. I'm on my way. I love you, Sis. I love you so much."

While I wait for Judy, I think about Dennis' last hospitalization and how scared Elizabeth was at the hospital. But will she be more scared if she sees him die at home? *God, where is the instruction book for this phase? How do I know what I'm supposed to do?* Since all the kids are home right now and Dennis is resting in the back, I decide to just tell them the situation and ask them what they want.

I round everyone up from the movie they're watching, and we all walk out to the back yard. I don't want Dennis to hear this conversation. "I think you all can see that Daddy is getting sicker, and I need you to think about something. Last time Daddy was in the hospital, it was a scary time for him. I would like to be able to keep him at home so that he doesn't have to go back to the hospital anymore. But you all live here, too, and maybe it makes you uncomfortable to see him so sick. I want you to think about this, and if you think you would feel better if Dad was in the hospital, all you have to do is tell me. We have to figure all this out as a family because it is not just Dad and me."

No one says anything for at least a couple of minutes, and then Drew asks, "If we say we want Dad in the hospital, then you'll just take him there?"

"No, I won't put him in the hospital unless he needs to go, but I will keep your request in mind as I decide whether or not to send him there. And you don't have to know right now what you want. This is a lot to think about so I need you to think about it for awhile."

No one has anything else to say right now, so we all walk back into the house, and the kids settle back down to finish their movie. Checking on Dennis, I can see he has fallen asleep so I decide it is a good time to wash a load of clothes.

Alice calls a little later, and when I tell her of my phone conversation with Donald, the response is immediate. "Joan, I'm on my way over, and I'm treating you all to pizza. Call the closest place to you all, and you and I will go get it when I get there."

Within twenty minutes, Alice has arrived, and we are headed to Domino's Pizza to pick up the order. "Okay, now exactly what did Donald say when you talked to him?"

"He said Dennis would be dead within a month."

"But what brought up the month? Was that because he quit taking the medicine or because you asked about Kathryn and school?"

"Because of Kathryn and school. That's why he said a month because I said Kathryn would leave in six weeks for school." I've somehow held it together all day—when I talked to Judy and when I talked to the kids, but now the reality is hitting me, and I begin to choke back the tears. "Alice, Dennis is really going to die. Really die. What in the world am I going to do?"

Without missing a beat, Alice stops the car, grabs my hands, and looks right into my eyes. "You are going to do what you've always done, Joan. You're going to take care of everyone. You're the one who has always done it, and you'll just keep doing it."

Mother calls later in the evening. Judy has called her, so she's calling to check on both Dennis and me. "Honey, I know Judy is coming tonight, but she does have to go home on Sunday, so I thought I'd drive up that afternoon."

"Of course, I would love to have you here, Mom, but you don't have to do that. We're doing okay; we really are."

"I know you're okay, Joan, but sometimes, if you don't have to be alone, you shouldn't be alone. And right now, you don't have to be alone. I know the kids are there with you, but you know what I'm talking about, Honey."

"I do, Mom, and thank you. I love you, and I'll see you Sunday. Please drive carefully. 'Bye."

"'Bye, Honey, I love you so much."

Judy arrives not long after I hang up the phone from Mother. She gives all the kids a hug, and, together, we walk back to the bedroom to see Dennis.

Dennis has drifted off to sleep, but somehow

he senses Judy's presence and opens his eyes almost as soon as she steps into the room.

Drowsily, "Is that my favorite sister-in-law I hear?"

"Your only sister-in-law, my friend. And yes, it is me, here to get your lazy butt out of bed. It's too early to go to bed."

"Gosh, it is good to see you. Come over here, sit by me, and give me a hug."

I leave Dennis and Judy alone and go back to clean up the remnants of the pizza. Judy and Dennis have long had a close relationship. She was just sixteen when we married, and Dennis was only too happy to have another little sister. Our own brothers were eight and eleven years older than Judy, so to have a big "brother" who, at twenty-one, was so close to her age and could share her music and understand her style of dress endeared Dennis to Judy. They need time together without anyone else around them.

Saturday seems to evaporate and, before I know it, it is time for dinner. Judy has offered to treat us to dinner out, but no one has any suggestions about where to go. Dennis is resting in the bedroom, so she walks back there to find out if he'll eat anything. "Dennis, if you could have anything in the world to eat tonight, what would you choose?"

"I don't know. I'm really not hungry."

"Oh come on, surely there is something that sounds good to you."

"Stuffed jalapeños from Ball's Hamburgers. Those sound good. And a bottle of champagne, too. That'll help wash 'em down, and I'll need a straw because then I won't have to sit up much."

"Stuffed jalapeños it is then."

"Don't forget the champagne," he calls out as we leave the room.

We get the orders from everyone else and check to see if anyone wants to go with us. No one else wants to ride, so I leave them all watching a movie and tell Elizabeth to check on her daddy in about ten minutes. Our order isn't quite ready when we get there, so I go into Albertson's and get Dennis a bottle of champagne and a box of straws. It may not interact well with the medicine that Donald sent, but he isn't keeping the medicine down anyway.

When we get home, Drew gets plates down and separates the burgers and the fries and dumps the jalapeños on another plate. Judy opens the champagne for me, and I stick a straw in the bottle. I grab a tray, put the plate of food and the bottle of champagne on the tray, and, together, we walk back to the bedroom. Dennis sits up, and I put the tray on the bed. He looks at the bottle of champagne, winks at me, and takes a sip through the straw. We all start laughing. He then picks up one of the jalapeños and takes a small bite. Judy and I each sit down at the end of the bed and begin our dinners.

Such a lovely evening, the three of us eating and laughing about things we've done over the

Just Keep Breathing

past twenty-four years. When Judy and I have finished our burgers, I leave the two of them alone and take our plates to the kitchen. Dennis has really eaten nothing. That first small bite he took from the stuffed jalapeños is all that is gone. I ask Samuel if he wants what is left of his dad's dinner, and he gladly takes them. Judy walks into the den and pulls Elizabeth and Drew into the kitchen with her to do the few dishes. Judy, rinsing out a Coke can, asks, "Where is your recycle container?"

"We don't recycle."

"You, you don't recycle!" Judy responds incredulously.

"No, what can I say. It's a Dennis thing. You know, you do all the work by rinsing and sorting the containers, then you take them to the recycle center, and the man there makes all the money." I add offhandedly, "When he's dead, I'll recycle."

After dinner, Judy and I take a short walk around the block. She has indicated the need to

170

talk to me. "Joan, what is Kathryn going to do about school?"

"She'll go back in August and finish. She has some scholarship money coming from Preston Hollow, and she's applied for enough financial aid for the year."

"Well, Marshall and I have talked about this, so here's what I want to do. As successful as I am, I still regret not finishing college. That's why I want to make sure that she has the money to finish this year. Whatever she lacks from the scholarships and financial aid, I will take care of for her. And this is a gift, Joan. I don't expect it to be repaid. You and Dennis mean everything to me, and I love Kathryn so much. Let me help in this way because there is nothing else I can do, but I can do this."

I can't help it. Before I can catch my breath, the tears are falling. Judy wraps me in her arms, and we stand in the middle of the street clutching each other for what seems like a lifetime.

The remainder of the evening is quiet. Judy has an early flight to catch, and the kids and I are all going to worship. Kathryn is being recognized as a scholarship recipient, and I want everyone there to support her. Dennis will be okay at home alone for a little while.

Sunday morning I get up early to kiss Judy good-bye. She doesn't want to wake Dennis, but I insist he would want her to wake him. After she hugs him and they exchange parting words, I walk her to the car. I assure her that I am okay, and she can go home. "We'll go to worship and see Kathryn get her scholarship. Mom will be here later this afternoon and that will be the most exciting thing that today entails. You go on and let me know when you're home. Thanks for coming up. You saved me this weekend; you really did. I love you."

"I love you." She backs out of the driveway and turns and waves one more time. "Remember how much I love you."

Dennis is fully awake when I walk back into the bedroom. A strange look on his face, I ask, "Honey, are you alright?"

"Scott, there's something going on in this room. It's like there's an aura or something. Do you feel it? It's there, and it's strange."

Kneeling beside the bed, I ask, "Dennis, do you think you're going to die soon?"

A moment of silence, then a single tear rolls down his face. He whispers, "Yes."

I immediately put my arms around him, and we hold each other for several minutes. Then he pushes away. "Scott, call my dad. I want Samuel, Drew, and Elizabeth to go there. They can't stay here. They can't."

"Dennis, are you sure? You want to send them to your dad's?

"Yes, I'm sure that's what I want to do. I can't tell them good-bye, Scott. I can't. Please call Dad."

Bob and Lil agree to come get Samuel, Drew, and Elizabeth and let them stay in Longview for the foreseeable future. They will come after church, and that gives me time to explain this to the kids and send them to church with Kathryn. I can't go now. I won't leave Dennis.

"Kathryn, come into the kitchen for a minute, please. I need to talk to you."

"What is it, Mom? Is something wrong?"

"No, I don't think so, but I can't leave Daddy this morning. Do you mind if I stay home with him, and you take Drew, Elizabeth, and Samuel with you? That way, you won't be alone when you get the scholarship."

"Sure, Mom, that's fine. Will you just help Elizabeth get ready so I can get ready?"

I ask Samuel, Drew, and Elizabeth to come into the den. "Bob and Lil are coming to get you all after church, and you're going back to Longview with them for a few days."

Samuel is quick to reply, "For how long, Mom? I don't want to go to Longview. Drew and Elizabeth can go."

"No, honey, I need you all to go. Daddy wants you all to go because he doesn't want you to see him any sicker. It'll just be for a few days, that's all."

"Okay, Mom. I'll do this because you asked, but I'd rather stay here."

A little while later, everyone is ready for church, and they come in to tell their dad and me good-bye. Drew, my hot-natured child, has put on shorts and a t-shirt. "Drew, you're going to worship, and shorts aren't really appropriate clothing for church," I remind him.

"Yeah, Drew, what are people gonna think if you show up in shorts?" Samuel cannot miss the opportunity to tease his little brother.

"Drew, little buddy, come here," Dennis has propped himself on his pillows and is motioning with his hand. Drew walks over to the side of the bed. "Son, you are such a smart young man. Remember that no matter what anyone else says, you know what's best for you. I love you so much and have always been so proud of you. You are going to be somebody really special. Don't ever forget that."

That is it for Drew as he collapses on his dad, sobbing. I get everyone out of the room, so the two of them can be alone. "Kathryn, Drew is going to stay home, but Samuel and Elizabeth will be there with you. I'll see you after worship. I love you."

Elizabeth wants to kiss her daddy good-bye, but I won't interrupt Drew's time with him. The crying has ceased, and they are sitting together on the bed talking. I walk the kids out to the car and then busy myself in the kitchen. Drew comes into the den about an hour and a half later. He sits down beside me and lifts my arm so he can snuggle close. Neither of us says a thing. He may only be eleven years old, but I know he'll remember the past two hours for as long as he lives.

"Mom, we saw Alice, and she asked why you weren't there." Kathryn, Samuel, and Elizabeth have arrived home from church. "I told her that Dad wasn't doing real well, and you didn't want to leave him. She said to call her if you needed something." I get Elizabeth to come help pack her bag because Bob and Lil will be here soon.

Shortly after lunch, Bob and Lil arrive and spend some time with Dennis. Samuel helps me put the bags in the car. Drew and Elizabeth hug Dennis good-bye, and Samuel follows them. As Samuel walks out of the room, he turns and looks at Dennis. "Are you sure you don't want me to stay and help here?"

Dennis shakes his head. "No, Son, we'll be fine. You help Dad and Lil with the kids."

"Okay, Dad. I, I'll see ya."

I assure all the kids that I'll call in a couple of days, and I thank Bob and Lil for coming. I watch them pull out of the driveway, and, as they turn the corner, I'm wondering what we're doing. Is this right, to send the kids away? I remind myself that this is what Dennis wants, so I just need to go with it and stop questioning.

I have to make him as comfortable as I can. Walking into the house, the silence hits me in the face. No television, no music, no voices. *Be still and know that I Am God.* I check on Dennis and find he's fallen asleep, so I sit on the couch and take a deep breath. I'm waiting. Right now, I'm waiting for Mother. I know I can't just sit and wait for things to happen, but, right now, Kathryn's gone to work, William is at his apartment, Samuel, Drew, and Elizabeth are on their way to Longview, and Dennis is asleep, and I am just going to sit here and be still for a little while. *Be still and know that I Am God.*

Mother arrives a little later in the afternoon. She looks good, but I can tell that she is so worried about me. "Honey, are you okay?" This strikes me as funny as soon as she asks the question. I am Joanie, the perennial happy and optimistic daughter who can always take care of herself.

Dennis is awake when we walk back to the bedroom. Mother and Dennis have shared such a special relationship. When she attempted to drive to Dallas for Mother's Day soon after my brother Scotty's brain damaging accident, Dennis is the one who drove one hundred miles east to pick her up when she decided she couldn't keep going. He stayed with her when Scotty died and helped her make the funeral arrangements in both Houston and Longview. After my father died and Mother decided to dispense with a Christmas tree, Dennis picked up the kids and me, and we took a Christmas tree to Mother's and then decorated it for her. Yes, they have a special relationship. She spends a little time with him and then comes in to sit with me in the den while Dennis naps.

The doorbell rings, and it is Sally Anderson, the mother of the young man whom Kathryn had been dating. Sally is a caterer and walks in with trays of food. "Joan, I didn't know what to do, but I had to do something. I thought, well, no matter what, people have to eat. I have a small ham, two roasted chickens, mashed potatoes, green beans, baked squash, sweet peas, chocolate chip cookies, and an apple pie. All you have to do is heat what you want."

"Gracious, Sally, I don't know what to say. You shouldn't have gone to this much trouble, really."

"It was no trouble at all, Joan. I love to cook; I had all the food at home; it just made me feel like I was doing something to help you because my heart is breaking for all of you. Now I'm going to get out of your way so you can continue to do whatever you were doing." We hug each other, and she is gone. I don't think she was in the house more than five minutes.

I put all the food in the refrigerator. Let's see, all this food for Mother, Kathryn, and me. No, I don't think we'll starve; that's for sure. Neither Mother nor I are hungry, but maybe Kathryn will eat a bite of something when she gets home from work. I know Sally thought everyone was home, and I didn't want to tell her that it was just the three of us. Truly, this food is a gift.

Monday morning Dennis wakes up with a little energy. "Hey, Scott, I want you to take me out to Restland."

"Okay, but why?"

"I want to pick out my burial plot, and I want to see if there is anything near Cora." Cora was Dennis' paternal grandmother and was the only person whom Dennis thought really loved him unconditionally. She died the fall before I met him.

"Okay, but I'm not sure walking around Restland is a good idea. I know I can rent a wheelchair at that pharmacy at Preston/Royal, so let me get dressed and I'll run get the wheel-chair. First, let me help you get showered and dressed."

"I can get a shower myself, but I do want you to stay in here with me just in case I start feeling whoozy."

While he showers, I gather his clothes and take them to the bathroom for him. As he steps out of the shower, I hand him a towel. I am horrified to see how skinny he is now. I know it hasn't happened overnight, but I think I've been going so fast, trying to keep all the plates spinning, that I just haven't noticed his weight. Now I see his rib bones, and his arms are like skin-covered bones with almost no tissue in between the skin and bone.

I leave him to dress and call Donald. "Donald, Dennis couldn't keep the medicine down, so he wouldn't even take it yesterday or today. He's not eating anything either."

"Joan, there's nothing else we can do. You asked me to tell you when it was time. It's time. There is nothing else to try. I'm going to call hospice for you. Is that okay?"

"How long, Donald? How long do we have?"

"Probably about two weeks. I can't say for sure, but I don't think he can last more than two weeks. The nurse from hospice will call you later and set up a time to come out. And, Joan, I'm really sorry. Call me anytime."

"Thank you, Donald. Thank you for everything." I hang up the phone, and I'm numb. I don't know what I expected Donald to say, but it wasn't this. Two weeks. Two weeks. Stop spinning world; I need some time. Two weeks.

CHAPTER 13

It is Over

Kathryn is home with Dennis, so Mother comes with me to run a couple of errands and get the wheelchair. I tell her what Donald says. "Joan, what are you doing about Dennis' funeral? You can't have the money for a funeral."

"No, Mom, I don't. I guess . . ." The tears start.

"Joan, honey, I'll pay for the funeral. Don't think about that at all. You've got so many people who love you, and you and Dennis have such wonderful children. You're going to get through this. You are."

We get to the pharmacy and get the wheelchair. By the time we get home, Dennis has already fallen asleep. He told Kathryn he was too tired to go to Restland; the shower drained him of all the energy he had.

It's lunchtime so Mother, Kathryn, and I walk to the kitchen and open the refrigerator door. All the food Sally brought overwhelms us, and I close the door immediately. I suggest to Kathryn and Mother that they go sit in the den, and I'll fix us some lunch. I slice some chicken and heat the potatoes. I know it is not a usual lunch for any of us, but nothing seems usual today.

"Mom, the phone's for you."

"Hello, this is Joan Curtis."

"Mrs. Curtis, this is Rachel with VistaCare Hospice Services. Dr. Donald Alexander called and said you are ready for hospice care."

"Yes, Ma'am, I am. My husband is terminally ill, and there is nothing left to do for him."

"Okay, if it's convenient for you, I'd like to send one of our nurses out tomorrow to meet with you and assess your husband's needs."

I make an appointment with hospice and then sit down and tell Kathryn what Donald Alexander told me that morning. One of the things I thought about after the kids left on Sunday was Dennis' mother. Even though Dennis had broken the relationship with his mother several years before, I knew I could not, as a mother myself, deny her the opportunity to tell her son good-bye. I call Mary, his mother, and then I call Sheila Jones. Sheila had been a business partner of Dennis for over fifteen years. I knew she would want to know. Kathryn and I spend some time talking about who else needs to be called.

Dale Andrews, a dear friend of Dennis, is standing on the step when I open the front door. Sheila has called Dale after she talked to me, and he is here to see Dennis. Walking back to the bedroom with Dale, I give him a quick summary of the situation. As soon as Dennis sees Dale, he sits up, and there is a big smile on his face. Dale walks over and takes his hand,

"Buddy, it is so good to see you." He shakes Dennis' hand, but he doesn't let go of it. I leave them alone, and I can hear them talking, and that's the most Dennis has talked all day. Dale comes into the den in about twenty minutes.

"Thank you for coming, Dale. I know how much that meant to Dennis. You made his day."

"It meant just as much to me, Joan. It made my day. Take care of yourself." He leaves, and I think he is the one real friend Dennis has. I'm so glad he came.

After Kathryn goes to work, I call Bob and Lil's so I can talk to the kids. Everyone is okay, but they are all worried about their dad. I try to calm their fears and remind them that this is what Daddy needs right now. Just hearing their voices—Elizabeth's smallness—Drew's huskiness—Samuel's tenderness—my heart breaks, and I have to stop listening and talk to myself so I can hold everything together enough to say good-bye. I promise to call again tomorrow and hang up the phone. After talking with them, I go back and lie down with Dennis. We don't talk; we just lie there together. Suddenly, I remember that Friday is July 13, and I know that Dennis will die on Friday. He's going to die on the thirteenth. I turn over, but he's asleep again. I stay next to him and will my heart to calm down.

Tuesday begins slow and quiet, but then begins the steady stream of people. About 11:00, Sheila Jones comes by to see Dennis. I explain that he's not always responding to what we say now, but he can carry on a short conversation before he gets too tired. I walk with her back to the bed-room and go in before her so that I can tell Dennis that she's here. He is really glad to see her. I leave them alone and go back in the den with Mother and Kathryn.

In about fifteen minutes, I hear Sheila's footsteps coming down the hall. She enters the room, and it is hard to describe the look on her face, not horrified but more disbelief. She grabs my hands, "Joan, I don't know what I was expecting, but, yes, I know what I was expecting. I was expecting him to be in his white dress shirt and tie. I know you said he was dying, and I know I was coming to say good-bye, but I still expected to find him in that damn white dress shirt and tie. I mean, that's Dennis." Now she's crying.

I put my arms around her. "You're right, Sheila, a white dress shirt and tie, that is Dennis. As recently as two weeks ago, he was worried about his hair being dirty when we went into Tom Thumb. But now, now he doesn't have it in him anymore."

Sheila hugs Kathryn and Mother good-bye, and I walk her to the car. Just as she drives out of the driveway, another car stops in front of the house. Getting out the car is a woman I don't know. We meet by the front steps, and I tell her who I am. "Hello, Mrs. Curtis, I am Helen with VistaCare Hospice. I will be your husband's nurse, but I am also here for you and your children."

"Hello, Helen. Please call me Joan, and let's go in and meet Dennis and our daughter Kathryn. My mother is also here with us."

Helen goes back to meet and assess Dennis. She already has the medical information, but she wants to be sure he doesn't need anything for pain or nausea or anything else. While she's back with Dennis, the doorbell rings. Kathryn answers the door and brings Dennis' mother and her two sisters into the den. Everyone hugs everyone else. We all talk for a few minutes, and when Helen comes back into the den, Kathryn takes Mary, Fern, and Dorothy back to Dennis. We shared such fun times with these women for most of the time we've been married. However, about six years ago, Dennis had enough of his mother's drinking to excess, and had let the relationship go astray. I know he is special to all these women, and this is going to be difficult for them.

Helen and I go into the living room to talk, so I can tell her about our family. In about ten minutes, Kathryn walks into the living room. "Mom, can I stay in here with you? They've all started crying, and I just can't stay back there any longer."

"Of course, Honey. Come sit here by me." She sits right next to me, legs touching mine. I put my hand on her leg and pat her softly. She looks at me, and we both start laughing. No words need to be said, but we both find it funny that she would choose to sit here discussing her father's impending death with the hospice nurse over being back with her wailing grandmother and great-aunts.

Everyone is here for another hour, and, by the time they all leave, I am exhausted. I go check on Dennis. I sit on the bed beside him and talk about the day. His eyes are open, but he doesn't say anything or make any acknowledgement that he hears me. William calls and says he'll be by tomorrow after work. A little later I can see that that Dennis has gone to sleep, so I go back into the den to sit with Mother. Kathryn is getting ready for work. I'm not really paying attention to what Mother is talking about, but I hear her say that the date today is July 11, and I realize that Friday is not the thirteenth, Thursday is the thirteenth. I breathe a sigh of relief. Dennis will not die on Friday.

Wednesday starts out hot. Of course, it's July in Texas so what else is it going to be. I call the kids at Bob and Lil's about mid-morning. They want to talk to their dad, but he's still asleep. We don't talk long because they are going to get a movie.

Dennis isn't really asleep, but he is getting more unresponsive. Kathryn and I noticed it yesterday, and we already see it today. Although it's still morning, and he slept through the night, we have no indication that he hears what we're saying. "Mom, do you think he hears us?" Kathryn is standing by me, and we're both right by Dennis lying in bed.

"I can't tell, Honey. I've knelt down beside him, but I can't even tell if I'm making eye contact with him. He just stares straight ahead. It's kind of eerie."

"Ya' know, Mom, he's probably just ignoring us. He's always been good at that, especially when it's the two of us talking to him." We both laugh, but it's an uneasy laugh.

Helen, the hospice nurse, comes by about 11:00. She's brought some medication to ease anxiety. "Helen, it is getting more difficult for Dennis to get to the bathroom. Could you catheterize him?"

"Mrs. Curtis, catheterization, although certainly appropriate in many cases, also increases the risk of infection. I'll have to call his doctor for an okay before I can do this procedure."

"Well, please call him today. It is humiliating to my husband for me to change his pants for him, and he doesn't have the strength to do it himself. In fact, you can call him from here because I need you to do this."

Helen steps over to the phone, pulls out her phone directory, and calls Donald. The conversation lasts about two minutes. As soon as Donald is put on the phone, he orders the catheterization without any hesitation. *Thank You, God, for leading us to Donald Alexander.*

"Mrs. Curtis, I don't have the supplies that I need for catheterization with me, but I will be back this afternoon and get this done."

"Thank you, Helen. I really appreciate this."

"The other thing I want to get you is a hospital bed."

"Oh, I don't want a hospital bed because I want Mr. Curtis in his own bed."

"And I understand that, but, as you've said, Mr. Curtis is getting weaker and weaker, and if he falls out of this bed, it can create even more problems for him and for you. Really, a hospital bed is for his protection and your peace of mind. I strongly recommend this for him."

"Okay, get the hospital bed. I'll trust you on this one."

"If I may use your phone again, I'll go ahead and order the bed. Then I'll go get the supplies

I need for the catheter, run by another patient's house, and be back here by mid-afternoon."

Helen leaves, and I try to get Kathryn to eat something. There is still so much food in the refrigerator because none of us has an appetite. Kathryn picks up a small piece of chicken and asks Mother if she can fix something for her. Mom accepts a small plate of food from Kathryn, and the two of them eat while I go back and lie down with Dennis. As has become usual now, we don't say anything, but I take his hand and hold it tightly while we lie in silence.

Alice drops by after lunch. She comes back to say hello to Dennis and me and then goes into the den and spends a little while talking with Mother and Kathryn. I can hear them laughing so that's good. Mother and Alice have always had a mutual affection for one another, so I'm glad they have this time together. And they are both such wonderful mentors for my dear Kathryn.

Helen doesn't get back with the catheter supplies until 2:30. She inserts the necessary tubing, and he's set. The hospital bed will be delivered in the morning. I decide to ask Helen about Dennis' unresponsiveness. "Helen, when we're talking to Dennis, we can't tell if he hears us because he doesn't give any kind of response. Do you think he hears us or what do you think is happening?"

"I can't say for sure, but my guess is that he's actually entered into the process of dying. If you've ever seen anyone coming out of a coma, it doesn't happen like on TV where it's like they're asleep and then bam, they're awake. When someone comes out of coma, it's a process, a slow process. They come back a little at a time."

"My brother was in a coma after a car accident, and that is how it happened. He came back in stages, where he was awake a little longer each day."

"Yes, well, what Dennis is doing is the opposite of coming back; he's going away a little at a time." As much as I hate thinking this, I do understand what she's saying. It makes sense.

After Helen leaves, my principal friend, Mary Steere, calls to see if she can stop by for a little while. She has been promoted from TJ and now works downtown but keeps tabs on the happenings at TJ. She arrives about 3:00, and after I catch her up on Dennis, she asks me about work. "You can't continue to support these kids on eleven thousand dollars a year. You need a teaching job."

"You're right, but it's not like I can go knock on doors asking for interviews right now."

"You don't need to do that. I happen to know that Cele Dominguez will be hiring people for TJ, so he needs to hire you. They'll take care of you at TJ. You're certified, aren't you?"

"Yes, I am."

"Okay, I'm going to call Cele right now." She picks up the phone and dials the number for TJ. "Cele, this is Mary Steere ... Yes, things are good with me. Don't you need a reading teacher for the fall? ... Well, I've got a teacher for you. Actually, it's Mrs. Curtis, the clerk who was taking care of the office the first part of the summer ... Yes, he is sick, but he's going die sooner than we thought, and she needs a job teaching, so she can support these kids ... Yes, she can do that, 10:00, she'll be there ... Thanks, Cele, you won't regret this.

"Okay, Joan, you've got an interview with Cele tomorrow at 10:00 at TJ. Go ahead and gather your paperwork for HR, but don't send it to them. Give it to Cele first, and then send copies to HR. They will lose your paperwork at least once, and that's why you want to always have what you need on campus in the hands of your principal."

"Thank you, Mary, thank you."

"Okay, let me talk to Kathryn for a little while and catch up with her. Let me know what happens tomorrow and call if you need anything. Anything at all."

Mary and Kathryn talk for awhile, and she leaves. All three of us are tired, so Kathryn offers a movie from Blockbusters. Mother and I can't be sure we'll stay awake through an entire movie. We decide to pick at some dinner and then just sit in front of the TV. At this point, none of us need our brains stimulated.

When I go back and check on Dennis, I hear something different with his breathing. It's like he's not breathing as deeply or something. "Kathryn, would you come back here for a minute?"

"Mom, what's wrong?"

"Listen to Daddy breathing. Do you hear something different?"

"Um, yeah, I do. It's like, it's almost like he's gasping, but he's not gasping."

"Like he's not breathing deeply; his breathing has become more shallow. I think that means he's getting closer, Kathryn." She comes to me, and we hold each other.

Thursday, July 13, 1995. The day seems almost surreal, as I plow through each minute, wondering what I will be doing the next minute and even when I interview for a teaching job in the morning, I am wondering what the afternoon will bring, never realizing the events are already in motion. When I get home from the interview, I go back to our bedroom and kneel beside Dennis. His eyes are open. "Honey, I have a job. Mr. Dominguez hired me to teach at TJ. I have a job so I can take care of us. Do you hear me, Dennis? It's okay now because we will be okay." I'm wondering if he understands me, so I lean over and kiss him. I feel his returning kiss; I know this time he hears me and understands me. He understands me.

The hospital bed has been delivered while I was gone, but I can't get Dennis to the bed. The bed is in our room, but Dennis has no strength, and I really think he's only partly still with us. He did return my kiss, but that was the first and only response in more than twenty-four hours. I don't want to leave Dennis, so Mother brings me a sandwich. She stays back here with me for a little while but then goes to answer the door.

Jan and Jim McBride are here. Jan and Jim are longtime friends from Longview. They moved in down the street from us when I was about twelve, and I used to babysit their children. Jan and Mother have been good friends all these years. They come back to see Dennis and me. Both Jan and Jim really want to see me because they know the situation, and they have always loved me. Jim asks about the hospital bed.

"Hospice ordered it, and it was delivered this morning, but I can't get Dennis to it, much less in it."

Jim, all of one hundred and fifty pounds, leans over and puts his arms under Dennis' neck and legs. "I'll carry him over there." He slowly picks him up and heads to the hospital bed.

I rush over and pull the sheet down, just as Jim gets there with Dennis. He lays him in the bed, and Dennis moves slightly. I skooch him over toward the middle and cover him with the sheet. "Thank you, Jim, thank you." I hug his neck, and then he, Jan, and Mother go back to the den.

I stay close to Dennis all day, listening as the breathing becomes shallower and shallower, almost wispy, and noticing, too, that Kathryn is walking back and forth, back and forth. I tell her to go to a movie because it could be hours before anything changes. She finally leaves about 8:30, and Mother walks back to check on me and then goes back outside to smoke a cigarette. Dennis' younger sister Diana has come, and I am not alone; Diana asks if she can stay with us and because I have lost my older brother, I know she needs to be here with her big brother. Each of us stands on either side of the bed, talking, laughing, crying, watching, listening for a change when suddenly his breathing is much slower, and I call Alice and manage to choke out, "Dennis is going to die soon so please say a prayer for us."

I go back over to Dennis, taking his hand, wiping his forehead, kissing him, reminding him, "I will always love you," and putting my head lightly on his chest, transferring all the love I feel for him into him, and I notice that there is no movement. I lift my head, listening, but hearing nothing, I look at Diana, saying, "He's not breathing," so she grabs my hand, and we listen harder, only stillness and absolute quiet, and we know. It is over. He is gone.

CHAPTER 14

Now What?

I'm not sure what to do first. I think I need to call hospice, so I walk over to the phone but then remember I need to tell Mother. Diana is just sitting on the bed, staring straight ahead, tears streaming. Mother calls hospice for me, so I just stand by Dennis. About ten minutes later, William is standing beside me and wraps me in his arms. A few minutes later, I ask him to get Kathryn. "She's at the movie; you know, over on Northwest Highway, that new one. I can't remember what she went to see. She just left about forty-five minutes ago. She's uh, uhm."

"It's okay, Mom. I'll find her and bring her home."

Within a few minutes, Helen from the hospice arrives and pronounces Dennis dead. She calls

Donald Alexander. "What funeral home are you using, Mrs. Curtis?"

"Restland, but I haven't made any arrangements. I, I didn't think it would be so fast."

"It's okay. I'll call them, and they'll come get him and take him to Restland. You can go tomorrow and make arrangements. It just saves you a step and some expense if they pick him up, and we don't need an autopsy, so there's no need to go to the hospital or morgue."

While Helen is on the phone, I'm wondering whether I should call the other kids. It's already 9:30, and I know Bob and Lil go to bed early. I don't know what to do. What's the right thing to do?

Mother has let Alice in, and she comes right back to the bedroom. Then Margaret is there because Diana has called her. I'm asking Alice about calling Bob, and Margaret says she's already called him, and they're bringing the kids home. Well, that's one decision I don't have to make. My dear friend Becky, who spent the evening with me in the hospital the week of her daughter's wedding, arrives shortly after Margaret; Alice called her. Becky and I meet Alice in the hall. "You have to help tell stories about him so Drew and Elizabeth don't forget him. But we will only tell the good stories." Becky smiles and puts out her arms. I fall into them, and Alice puts her arms around us, too. "They are so little. What am I going to do?"

Finally, William is home with Kathryn. I'm standing by the bed, with Dennis, and I turn to take her in my arms. My heart hurts so much for her, for William. It really hurts. I can't think about me yet because I'm too worried about how to tell Samuel, Drew, and Elizabeth. Or will Bob have already told them?

Restland calls to say they are on the way to pick up Dennis. I want some time with him before they take him away. I ask Mother to take Kathryn into the den, and William, Becky, Alice, Diana, and Margaret all follow.

I don't say anything. I just sit on the bed and hold his hand and remember. I remember the day I met him and thought he was so cute. I remember the day he asked me to marry him, and I had to ask him if that's what he was asking. I remember the day I told him I was pregnant with Kathryn, and we went to El Chico's in Inwood Village to celebrate, and I had two glasses of milk. I remember asking him what if Scotty was really hurt, and my parents couldn't take care of him, and Dennis just said we'd bring him to our house. I remember the three of us—Mother, Dennis, and me—being with Daddy in his hospital room when Daddy stopped breathing. I'm not sure who hurt more at that moment—Mother, Dennis, or me. I remember the day my world stopped when he told me he had AIDS. And now—now all of our life together is just a memory.

I open the door, and there are a man and woman in the hall, both from Restland. I introduce myself, show them Dennis, and they go to work. Somehow they wrap him in sheets and move him to their stretcher. Then they wheel him out to the hearse. The whole process seems like it only takes about thirty minutes. I feel like this is all a dream.

My principal friend Mary has arrived while the people from Restland are getting Dennis ready. She now gets everyone moving. "Joan, do you want the medicine and everything out of your room?"

"Yes, let's get all that stuff out before the kids get home. I don't want them to see any trace of illness." Everyone jumps up and goes to the bedroom to grab something. Anything to feel like they're doing something to help. Medicine is put in a drawer. Sheets are removed from the bed and put in the hamper. Bed is folded, and bed and potty chair and oxygen tank are put in the garage. Mattress pads, latex gloves, water pitcher, and drinking glass are all put in a lower cabinet in the bathroom. Within twenty minutes, there is not one sign that anyone in the house was sick.

Finally, we hear the car outside, and I know the kids are home. I walk out the door, followed by Kathryn, William, and Mother. Samuel is the first one out of the car, so he is the first one in my arms. "He's gone, Honey. It was all very peaceful, just a slowing down of the breathing until he stopped. He loved you so much, Samuel." He can't say anything for a minute.

Finally, I hear, "I know, Mom."

Kathryn has Drew, so I take Elizabeth and walk with her into the house. We sit on the sofa in the living room. I don't even know what to say. She's only seven years old. "Elizabeth, Daddy died tonight, so that means he isn't sick anymore. We won't get to see him, and we'll really miss him, but at least we know he isn't sick anymore. And he loved you so much."

"Daddy's gone forever, Mommy?"

"Yes, Sweetheart, he's gone forever until we see him in Heaven when we die. But we'll still feel him in our hearts, and we'll remember all the good times we had and that's how we'll keep him with us."

"Can I see him?"

"No, the doctor has already taken him away."

By now everyone has come back in, so Mother comes in to take Elizabeth while I go find Drew. "Kathryn told me, Momma. Daddy died."

"Yes, he did. He loved you so much, Drew, and I'm so glad you had that time with him on Sunday." I take him in my arms, and he holds on as if he's holding on for dear life. *God, please help me. Please help me help my children. If ever I could do the right thing, let it be now. Please, God, please help me.*

"Where is he, Momma? Where's all the stuff?"

"The people from the funeral home have taken him to get him ready for the funeral we'll have, and all the medicine and the portable potty and the oxygen tank are in the garage. No one is sick anymore, so we don't need all that in the house."

We all gather in the den. Mother, Alice, Becky, Mary, Diana, Margaret, William, Kathryn, Samuel, Drew, Elizabeth, and I sit in chairs and on the couch where everyone is touching someone else. I look around me and see my family of blood and my family of heart. It all seems so surreal.

"Thank you all for helping me take care of Dennis," I say to everyone, looking around the room. I look at our kids, "Your daddy. He loved you all so much. Mother, he knew that you were a more loving mother to him than his own mother. I know you were his little sisters, Diana and Margaret, but he loved you both almost as a parent. He always wanted to protect you both. Alice, Becky, and Mary, he knew what good friends you are to me. In fact, I think he only knew one friendship like the ones I share with the three of you. That's why he could understand and why he didn't let himself worry too much about me. He knew you all would take care of me."

I take in the faces of our children. "He couldn't have loved you all more if he tried. He was so proud of you all. I want you to remember all the good times we had—the LaffyTaffy jokes driving home from Herrera's, all the drives to have brunch when we heard 'smile on your face and song in your heart.' Remember how much we all wanted to hit him then?" I see small smiles on all five faces. "Just don't ever forget how much he loved you. Now it is very late, and I think it would be good if we all tried to get some sleep. The next two days will be busy."

"Mommy, can I sleep with you?"

"Yes, Sweet Pea. I'm not going to bed right now, but I'll tuck you in and be there in a little while."

Alice, Becky, and Mary leave with promises to be back first thing in the morning, and I then go back in to see that the kids are getting undressed. I offer a bed to William, but he decides to go to his apartment. "I think I'll sleep better there, Mom. I'll be back in the morning. I love you."

"I love you, too, Honey. We will get through this, okay?" I hug him tightly.

It is 12:30 a.m. now, so we have already moved past the 13th. Today is Friday, July 14th. I go in and kiss Samuel good-night, then go to Drew and tuck him in tightly and kiss him good-night. Kathryn is in her room reading so I go to my room and lie down with Elizabeth in my bed. I pull her close to me and stay there until she is asleep. I get up and go into Kathryn's room and sit down on the side of her bed. We don't talk; we are there together, tears falling silently. I just want to take the pain away from all of them, but I know I can't. Surely, this is the most difficult thing I have ever faced as a mother. I can't do anything to help them; their father is dead; my husband is dead. Life is forever changed.

Kathryn finally falls asleep. I move Elizabeth to her bed because I don't know how well I'll sleep, and I want Elizabeth to sleep as long as she can. I finally get in the bed about 3:00 a.m., and the last time I see the clock, it is 3:30.

I wake with a start at 5:30 a.m. The events of the last twelve hours wash over me, and I just want to go home. Although we are here together in this rental house, it is not our home. Our home is the house at 10244 Hedgeway. The house where we have reared our children, where we have hunted Easter eggs and had wonderful Thanksgiving and Christmas Dinners. That's where I want to be—home. I throw on some shorts and a t-shirt, tiptoe down the hall to get my keys, and ease out the front door.

There's only one car in the driveway—my car. Where's Kathryn's car? I shut my eyes and open them again. One car. Oh! Maybe Kathryn got up and wanted to go home, too. We are so much alike. I quietly open the door and go back to the girls' room. Gently, I peek in expecting only Elizabeth, but there's Kathryn, too. She didn't take her car.

I go back outside and walk to the back of the house. Maybe she parked back there, but there's no car, just like I knew there wouldn't be. I sit down on the front steps. I don't understand. Where is Kathryn's car? Head in my hands, tee shirt already starting to stick to my back from the Texas heat, the conversation starts in my head. I know God wouldn't let Dennis die, and Kathryn's car be stolen in the same night. *Joan, God doesn't work like that.* I know God doesn't work like that, but if He did, I know He wouldn't let Dennis die and Kathryn's car be stolen in the same night. *He doesn't work like that, Joan. There is an explanation*, but what is it?

I don't understand what's going on, but I get in my car and drive home to Hedgeway. The house is warm but not hot. The air conditioner is on because my friends have been painting the rooms for us. I walk through slowly. It's looking good, but we're not quite ready. I had hoped to be able to move Dennis back here before—well, we didn't make it.

I walk back outside and look at the pool. It doesn't look good, but I can't worry about that now. I head down the driveway to the front yard and see two neighbors on their daily run. Edna Clemens and Betty Cree see me and stop to say hello.

"Hi, Edna. Hi, Betty. I have to tell you that Dennis died last night."

They are both so shocked they're at a loss for words. "Joan, I am so sorry," Edna finally manages to get her breath.

"Me, too," Betty adds. "Had you already made any arrangements?" They knew he was sick.

"No, not yet. I didn't expect this to happen this soon even though I knew it was coming. I'll go to Restland today, and something will be in the paper later. I have to get back over to the other house now because I want to make sure I'm there when the kids wake up. It's good to see you both."

Both women walk over and hug me, and then they are back on the street heading home. I watch them for a few minutes and then I'm back in the car headed to Thunder Road. As soon as I pull in the driveway, I realize that Kathryn's car is at the theater. Of course, William picked her up and drove her home.

No one is awake, so I lie down on the couch until I hear footsteps in the hall. Kathryn is the first one up, followed closely by Drew, Samuel, and, finally, Elizabeth and Mother. I fix some breakfast and make an appointment with Restland for 10:30. Libby Flory calls and asks if it would help to have Elizabeth come over and play with Hannah. Libby and Mark Flory and their three daughters are some of the nicest people I know. I can't think of a better place for Elizabeth to spend the day. Suma Napper then calls about Drew—the Napper boys want him there—Suma, Jon, and the four boys want him there because they love him as if he's the fifth son. I don't know if this is the right thing to do—send Elizabeth with Hannah's family and Drew with the Nappers, but I have so much I have to do today, and they are both so young and don't need to do these things. I'm really grateful to have the Nappers and the Florys to love and nurture my children on this day.

Mother, Kathryn, and I will go to Restland, and, after lunch, we'll go to Preston Hollow Presbyterian Church to meet with the associate minister. Blair Monie, the senior pastor, is out of town. I'm really disappointed, but, in the long run, I don't guess it really matters. I do confirm with the church that we can have a memorial service on Saturday early in the afternoon. It's mid-July in Texas; I have to think about people in the heat. We will have a small graveside service in the morning with family and then go to the church where there will be a focus on the resurrection and our continuing life in God. That is what I need to hear and what I want our children to hear.

Mother, Kathryn, and I are sitting in a receiving room at Restland Funeral Home. We've already picked out the coffin and the burial plot; it is across the street in a new development. I laugh with Kathryn about this being the perfect place for her dad because he'd soon be talking about the potential in this new area. He was such a visionary and could see real potential in ideas I thought were crazy or impractical and in houses that horrified me. Our first house had torn carpet, stained walls, and a repugnant smell. He had bargained with the owner, a sixty-something woman (we thought "old" woman because we were twenty-one), that if she would lower the rent and buy the paint, we would paint the interior ourselves. She had also agreed to replace the carpet. Dennis had been so excited, and I had cried because I didn't want Mother to see where I was living. He had been right; it had turned out to be a really cute first house, and I had cried when we moved out of it.

"We want a double plot in that section," Mother says to the director.

"Mother, I don't have to have a double plot now."

"I know, Honey, but let's go ahead and get a double plot and then you don't have to think about that again or worry that someone else will buy that piece, and you can't get it."

"Okay, if you're sure, Mom."

"I can do this so let me do this," she assures me.

"What about visitation? Since your service is in the morning, do you want to have visitation hours this afternoon or this evening for people to pay their respects and say good-bye?" The director is talking to me.

"No, his death is not sudden, and people who needed to say good-bye have already done that." I'm not looking at Kathryn or Mother. This is my decision, and I feel strongly about this. "He had lost so much weight, and I don't want people to remember him like that." Sheila's reaction on Tuesday is influencing my decision. She wanted to remember him in his white dress shirt and tie. "I don't want the coffin opened for anyone." I look at Kathryn. "Do you want to see Dad again? Do you think the other kids should see him again?"

"No, Mom, I don't want to see him, and I don't think they should see him either. Let us remember him alive and being funny or irritating."

"Okay, then I do not want his coffin opened for anyone."

"Yes, ma'am. Do you want to use our car services? Since you are starting at the burial site in the morning and then going to the church, we won't be transporting the body anywhere, so you don't really need our limousines unless you want them."

"No, we don't need the limousines. That's just needless expense." I look at Mom.

"That's fine, Honey, if you don't want to use their car services. Certainly, you have enough drivers in your family. But don't think about the money. Do what you want because I don't want you to have any regrets later," Mother is holding my hands as she talks. I don't know what I would do if she weren't here with me.

"Let's see what we have now," the director begins going over the list. "We'll close the coffin today, and see you all at 10:30 in the morning at the graveside. We'll have a tent and a few chairs, and two of our attendants will be there. Your minister will conduct a short service. Do you want any flowers from us?"

"Yes, I would like two sprays, one from Joan and her children and one from me," Mother tells the director. "And no carnations in either spray."

"We can do that," he responds. He quickly adds everything. "With the obituary for the paper, death certificate copies, that comes to $13,729.72 total."

"Thirteen thousand dollars?" I don't hear the other numbers because I am horrified!

"Joan, it's okay. It's okay," Mom grabs my hands again and looks at the director, "Is a personal check okay?"

"Yes, Ma'am, perfectly okay. Now is there anything you want to put in the coffin with him before we seal it and what do you want on the gravestone? Dates of birth and death? Just the years? Your name and his?"

Kathryn quickly responds, "Mom, please don't put your name on the stone. It'll be hard enough for us to see Daddy's; we don't want to think about you dying, too."

I look at the director, "Just his name, but I want full dates, not just the years. *Dennis Mark Curtis, January 29, 1951 to July 13, 1995*. I also have his wedding ring. He took it off when the weight loss meant it didn't fit, but I'd like you to put it back on his finger." I start to hand him the ring when Mother puts her hand on mine.

"I remember Mom giving me my father's wedding ring when he died. It kept him close to me for a long time." My mother had lost her father when she was nineteen, just a year younger than Kathryn.

"Kathryn, this isn't the ring I gave your daddy when we married because that one was stolen when he was mugged, but do you want this one? He did wear this one for several years."

"Thank you, Mom. I do want it." I hand it to her and keep her hand in mine.

"Then I think we're through here," I look at the director. "Thank you for everything."

"We will have everything ready for you tomorrow morning. Do not hesitate to call if you think of anything else."

"Okay. Please wait to seal the coffin. I don't think I want to come back, but I'm not ready to close that door yet."

"We'll wait until the morning. You come back at any time before then if you want to," he has my hands and is looking right into my eyes.

"Thank you. Thank you for everything."

Later that afternoon, Samuel hears me talking on the phone. "We're all in a bit of a shock, but at least we know he's not sick anymore, and that's a good thing."

"That's no comfort for me," Samuel comments, not looking at me. "I'd take him back in a second; I don't care if he's sick; I just want him here."

I hang up the phone and go sit down beside him and take him in my arms. "I know, Honey, I know. I'm just saying what people want to hear. It makes them feel less helpless if they think we're doing okay. Right now, I don't know if I'll ever be okay again."

We all go to the church to meet the minister and tell him about Dennis. I have chosen the hymns I want to sing and the scripture I want to hear. He will add other scripture, and the church will provide food for a reception after the service. Since Blair is out of town, I had asked Sally Brown if she would do the service. Before she had gotten her divinity degree, she had been the Director of Children's Christian Education at Preston Hollow, and I have known her for years. Even though Dennis didn't go to church, Sally had watched our older kids grow up, so I just felt she knew us and would do a better job at the memorial service. But as a current minister at NorthPark Presbyterian Church, she could not take precedence over the minister who does have a position at Preston Hollow, so she agreed to read scripture. At least that way, someone will be up there who knew us before today.

Judy, Marshall, and my nephew Bryan have arrived by the time we get home. Judy and I fall into each other's arms, and we both fall apart—but only for a minute. I give them the update on the services, and we talk for just a few more minutes before they leave to check into a hotel that's close. I feel better just knowing that they're here, and I know Mother feels better, too.

I hear Kathryn on the phone in the kitchen. "I'm scheduled to work tomorrow, but my father died last night, and the funeral is tomorrow. I'll be in at the regular time on Sunday." Kathryn quit her job with Olive Garden and now waits tables at Uncle Julio's at Frankford and the Toll-way. Are they really going to ask her to work on Sunday, three days after her father died? "Thank you. I will do that, and I'll call on Monday to find out when I'm scheduled to work for next week. I really appreciate this." She hangs up the phone.

"Are they giving you Sunday off?" I ask her, being careful not to put much *surely they are* in my voice.

"Yes, Mom, I don't have to work Sunday or Monday, and they said they'd keep me off the schedule next week, too, if I want them to. I'll see how I feel on Monday. It might be that working is good for me right now, and I do need as much money as I can make before I go back to school."

Mother encourages me to lie down for awhile, and I do just that. Two hours of sleep are not going to get me through the next few days. I manage to doze for a little while and then hear the doorbell. I make myself get up and hear my brother's voice as I head to the den. Arthur is here. I never thought he would come, but I should have known he would. Mother, Judy, and Arthur—I am so glad they're all here with me.

Saturday morning Kathryn comes into my bedroom. "Mom, Samuel says he's not going to Dad's service."

"Thank you, Honey. I'll go talk to him. But I can't make him go. He has to make the decision for himself."

Samuel is sitting on his bed in his room. I sit beside him and take his hand. "Samuel, I'm not going to tell you that you have to go to Dad's funeral. I can't even imagine how this must be for any of you. I lost my dad when I was thirty-three and thought that was too young. So I'm not even going to try to make you go. I will say you can wear anything you want—even that awful port-a-pit (portable track sand pits) t-shirt—anything that you will be comfortable in. And you don't have to stay at the church after the service and talk to people. You all can come straight home. And the last thing I want to say is that if you choose not to go, I believe that someday, maybe ten or twenty or thirty years from now, you will wish that you had gone.

Well, that's the second to last. The last thing is that I love you and nothing will ever change that." I kiss him on his forehead and leave him to make his own decision.

We limit the graveside services to family and the closest of friends. We arrive about 10:20. Of course, Alice is there when we arrive, as are Becky and Dave. It is all so unreal that I am not even certain of whom I do see. I know Dennis' mother Mary is there, as are his sisters Margaret and Diana and their husbands Roy and Tom. Bryant, his brother is there, too. Dennis' aunts, Fern and Dorothy, are with his cousin, Carolyn, and her husband, John. The rest, Judy, Marshall, and Bryan are here with my brother, Arthur. Arthur has driven the car with Drew, Elizabeth, Mother, and me. There are four chairs on each row so I sit between Drew and Elizabeth, and Mother sits beside Elizabeth. Kathryn, Samuel, and William sit behind us. The minister is talking, but all I can hear is Elizabeth's little voice. "Daddy, don't be dead. Please don't be dead."

Sounds of light laughter from behind, and I know Kathryn is doing whatever she has to do to keep Samuel together. If they laugh through their father's funeral service, so be it. I can't even think about what this means for me because right now I just wish I could take the pain away from our children. Drew is crying now, taking gulps of air. I pull him close.

I hear scripture and now we're getting up. I turn around and thank everyone, take Drew and Elizabeth's hands and head to the car, remembering that I just have to put one foot in front of the other and take one step at a time. Drew and Elizabeth are both crying so hard now, and I don't seem to be able to say anything so I just squeeze their hands tighter. *I can't do this, God. You have so misjudged me because I can't do this. I can't.*

All of a sudden, my knees start to give, and I feel myself going down slowly. Almost simultaneously, Dave Neeley is behind me with his hands under my elbows, lifting me up. He leans forward and puts his mouth right next to my ear. "Just keep breathing, Joan. Just keep breathing."

CHAPTER 15

Closure Does Not Begin on Monday

As we leave the cemetery, my mind is scrambling. I can't give in now. Just keep breathing, Joan; just keep breathing. Drew and Elizabeth are both settling down some. Elizabeth has her head in my lap. Drew is holding my free hand and looking out the window. Although we are going right to the church, we don't have to hurry. I don't want either of them to deny or bury their sadness, but we still have to get through the memorial service, and it will be easier for me if they're not hysterical. "I know; let's stop and get a Slurpee. We can stop at Daddy's favorite 7-11 because it's right on the way to the church. Would you all like to do that?"

Elizabeth perks up a little. "I want a cherry Slurpee, Mommy."

"Okay, Sweet Pea, then a cherry Slurpee it is. Driver, to the 7-11 at Preston and Royal, please."

Arthur responds, "Yes, Ma'am. Right away, Ma'am."

"You're funny, Arthur," Elizabeth tells her uncle, and she's smiling when she says it.

We stop at 7-11 and get our Slurpees. They do taste good on this hot summer morning. Upon arriving at the church, Elizabeth hands me her cup to throw away. Of course, the top is loose, and, in trying to balance it with my cup and purse, I spill the cherry liquid down the front of my white blouse.

We are early, but we don't have time for me to go home and change. I don't care. Dennis is dead. I'm at his funeral. Does it really matter that I have cherry Slurpee on the front of me? We walk into church, and I see Jeanne Harvey, my colleague from Good Shepherd. Jeanne hugs me but then sees the red stain on my blouse. "Joan, what happened? You can't go in there like that."

"Jeanne, it doesn't matter. I mean, in the grand scheme of things, what does a little Slurpee stain matter?"

"I know, Joan, I know. But you don't want to look like this for Dennis' service. Let's go to the bathroom and switch. You can wear my gold blouse, and I'll wear the white blouse with Slurpee on the front."

I agree, and we head to the nearest restroom. I put on Jeanne's blouse, and she puts on mine. As soon as I look at her, I'm laughing. "Jeanne, the stain looks fine, but your black bra underneath that white blouse is a real eye catcher."

"Oh, crap. I forgot about that. Okay, let me have my gold blouse back, and I'm going to go find someone to change with you." She puts her blouse back on and heads down to the sanctuary. I can't believe I'm at my husband's funeral and am waiting in the bathroom while a friend finds someone to change clothes with me. The absurdity of the whole situation is more than overwhelming.

In about ten minutes, Patrice Dormen comes through the bathroom door, followed closely by Jeanne. "I understand you need a blouse without Slurpee stains. I think this one will do." Without a moment's hesitation, she is removing her blouse and handing it to me. "The best part of your blouse, Joan, is that I can wear it backwards, and this lightweight jacket will cover up the stain." She gives me a quick hug and is gone before I get her blouse on; I seem to be moving in slow motion.

The service is okay. We asked the minister to talk about the visionary that Dennis was and the father and husband. The hymns are beautiful, and I could have chosen more. I remember when my brother, Scotty, had his car accident and was critically brain damaged, I wouldn't sing in church because I was so mad at God. I'm not mad now. I understand that God is not doing this, but He is going to help us get through it. I don't know why it is happening; I'm lost, I'm confused, I'm sad, I'm scared, but I'm not mad.

After the service, we leave the sanctuary and stop to accept people's condolences. Mother, Kathryn, William, and I are standing so people can see us. Arthur comes to tell me that he is taking the other kids home; they want to leave. I give my okay; I'm glad he's there to take them.

A young woman approaches and calls my name. I do not know her. "Joan, I'm Cyndy Monie, Blair's wife. He is out of town and called and asked me to come. He is deeply sorry that he's not here."

"How do you do, Cyndy. I really appreciate your coming today. I know it can't be easy to go to a funeral when you don't know anyone. Thank you and thank Blair."

I look past Cyndy Monie and can't believe the two people walking up to me. Patti Machin-Garrett and her mother, Clara Machin. Patti and I have been close friends since we were ten years old and in fourth grade. She and Gary moved to Tennessee in 1974, but Patti and I have stayed in contact with each other so that our friendship did not fall by the wayside.

"Patti, what are you doing here? How did you know?"

She wraps me in her arms. "I was planning a trip to Texas to see Mother this weekend, but Tuesday I told Gary I needed to leave the next day because something told me that I needed to already be here by the weekend. Someone called Mother yesterday so I knew."

"Please come by the house, Patti. You can do that, can't you?"

"Yes, we'll come to the house. I'll get the address from William."

It seems like we stand here for hours and talk to people, but I know it only seems that way. Kathryn, William, Mother, and I finally leave and head home. The house is full of people, but I spend most of the time with Patti. Somehow it means so much to have someone here who has always known me and shared the days of dating and falling in love with Dennis. Patti was in our wedding, just as I was in hers. I will never forget that she and her mother came here today.

Somehow the hours pass, and we all manage to get through this day. I had hoped to get Dennis home to Hedgeway, but it didn't happen. We are moving home next Saturday, and we will go home without Dennis. I don't want to think about that now. Finally, it is night, and everyone has gone to bed. I think I can even sleep tonight.

Sunday morning Becky calls to see if I want to go to church with Dave and her. I know it is too much to ask the kids to go, and I don't want to go by myself, but I know being surrounded by people of faith will be good for me. I decide I do want to go with them.

Becky and Dave pick me up about 10:30 and as we pull out onto the street, Dave asks, "Becky, did you tell Joan about our miracle yesterday?"

"My gosh, what happened?" Even as numb as I feel, I am curious.

"We left the cemetery and stopped at McDonald's at Preston/Royal. It was so hot, and we knew we had time to sit and relax for a few minutes. You won't believe this, but when we got back in the car, Dave couldn't get the motor to start. He tried over and over, for about ten minutes, but, by then, he had used what battery there was. We actually thought, no big deal, we can walk because it's just up Preston to Walnut Hill."

"Becky, that's a mile! Did you not realize that?"

"We realized it quickly once we started walking. Dave had on his coat and tie, and I had on heels, and it must have been 110 degrees. Anyway, we walked about two blocks and got to St. Mark's, and you won't believe this, but a cab stopped, and the driver asked if we wanted a ride."

"Cab? You mean a taxi? There was a taxi on Preston Road?"

"Yes, have you ever seen a taxi on Preston, especially there by Royal and Walnut Hill?"

"No, never, not in my twenty-three years of living here."

"Well, that's why Dave refers to it as our miracle. What else could it be?"

"I guess that's it. A miracle. Dave, what car are we in now? I'm not going to chance another miracle today in the form of cab on Preston in case we get stuck."

"It's okay, Joan. We're in a different car so we'll get you to church and home again with no problem."

Church is good. It is good to be with others who share my faith. People are compassionate and kind. The hymns bring tears and resolve that, with God's help, I will get through this. I love Becky and Dave and feel safe with them.

When I get home, Judy and Kathryn are fixing lunch for people. As we eat, Judy comments that she and Marshall have talked and agreed that she and Bryan will head back this afternoon, but Marshall will stay here and help get the house on Hedgeway ready for us to move back. Being optimistic, I had set a moving date of July 22, believing that Dennis would be going home with us. Alice had worked hard to get our bedroom ready for Dennis, but, of course, it won't be happening as I thought it would. We'll finish the few things that still need to be done this week, and we'll keep the moving date of next Saturday.

Mother offers to take Elizabeth home with her for a few days. I know that will help me. I can concentrate on helping on Hedgeway. Elizabeth doesn't really want to go, but I explain that I will be busy and can't stay with her, and it will only be for three days. I will get her on Wednesday, and we'll move back into our house on Saturday. Knowing that she's going home is enough, and she leaves the table to pack a bag for "Dear's house."

After lunch, Judy is standing at the kitchen sink. She turns around with a Coke can in her hand, looks at me, and asks, "Where's your recycle container?"

Instantly I am back at her same question only one week ago, and I am remembering my response. "When Dennis is dead, I'll recycle." I wonder if Judy remembers our conversation last week, and this is her attempt at humor or if she does not even remember last weekend. I suppose many people would consider this sick humor, but I think Judy remembers, and she is letting me know that we will laugh again. Maybe not now, but it will happen. We will laugh.

By late afternoon, Mother has left with Elizabeth, and Judy has left with Bryan. Kathryn has gone back to her room to lie down for a while, and Marshall has gone over to Hedgeway to see what's left to be done. Samuel, Drew, and I are sitting together in the den and mostly just silent. I think we are all emotionally spent and numb. Samuel finds a movie, puts it on, and we all sit and stare at the television.

Monday morning the phone rings. "Hello."

"May I speak to Joan Curtis?" I do not recognize this voice.

"This is she. Who's calling?"

"Mrs. Curtis, this is Cele Dominguez, TJ principal. I talked with you last Thursday and said we could hire you to teach reading. Well, I just got word from our human resources department that they have hired all the reading teachers needed and will be sending one out to Thomas Jefferson. I'm sorry, but I don't have a job to offer you now."

My response is automatic, as if I am on remote. "Okay. Thank you for calling, Mr. Dominguez." I hang the phone up and turn around to see Kathryn. "I guess it's too late to tell Daddy not to die. That was Mr. Dominguez, and I don't have a job after all. I don't know how I'm going to take care of everyone."

CHAPTER 16

One Step at a Time

Tuesday morning I meet Marshall, Alice, and Becky at our house on Hedgeway. We spend the day painting the den. I can't help but think how happy Dennis would be now. The people renting the house had painted all the rooms in quite vivid colors—bright blue, shiny gold, lime green, pumpkin orange—but once we finish the den, the house will be off white once more. I always teased Dennis that paint did come in colors other than white and off white.

By 5:00 we are all starving, so Alice volunteers to make a Whataburger trip. Hamburgers sound good to all of us so while she makes the food run, Becky and I clean paint brushes. Another room finished; we are almost there.

We sit on the floor in the den to eat. Everybody is tired, but relaxed, and the food is just what we needed. I'm explaining what happened to the teaching job when Marshall asks if there is anything else I want to do. Suddenly I realize that I can do anything I want to do because my reason for entering the world of education was insurance for Dennis, and now I don't need that. Oh my word, there is light at the end of the tunnel! I can't help it—I start laughing. Real, gut felt laughter. *We're going to be okay, aren't we, God? You're not going to let us stay down. We are going through the valley, not taking up permanent residence.*

Wednesday evening I run by Hedgeway to drop off a box from the garage at the rented house. I see Samuel in the den as I pull into the driveway and drive to the back of the house. When I open the back door, which opens into the den, I see Samuel. Hammer in one hand, nail and framed picture in the other, he is studying a photo he has taped to the wall. The tears form in my eyes. This wall in the den is twenty feet wide, and Dennis and I had been hanging 5" x 7" pictures of the kids in clear plastic frames for the past eighteen years of living in this house together. When we moved to Virginia, over one hundred framed pictures had been packed in a box and never unpacked. Until now. Samuel is studying a photo previously taken in the den so that he can get the framed pictures hung where they had been before moving. What Samuel is really doing is attempting to make our house on Hedgeway—our home—look like we never left it so that we can pretend that nothing has changed. But everything has changed and some-how we are all going to have to find a way to live with the changes.

Early Saturday morning, people show up from everywhere to take a load of clothes, boxes, small furniture—I can't even count all the peo-ple who are here to help us. Judy has come back, and it helps just to know that she's here with me. Dennis' brother Bryant has come and brought friends to help him move the bigger furniture. Drew and Elizabeth get in my car, and we head over to Hedgeway. They are both excited to be home and quite willingly take charge of their things to begin putting them back in their rooms.

Standing in the kitchen, someone asks where the pots go. I'm trying to think where I kept them, but, honestly, I don't even care where they go. I look at the spot for the refrigerator and wonder how Bryant and his friends are going to move it. Before I can figure it out, Judy and Becky approach me together. "Joan, can we talk with you outside for a minute?" Judy asks.

"Sure, is something wrong?"

"Yes and no, but we've got a solution so that's what we need to discuss."

When we get outside, Judy and Becky tell me that my refrigerator is old, and the seal for the door is torn and cannot be replaced. Marshall has already looked into it. Then I hear words from Becky that I have trouble processing right away.

"Joan, Dave and I have talked about this with Judy and Marshall, and we want to buy you a new refrigerator. Will you let us do that?"

"You want to buy me a new refrigerator? But why?"

"Well, there are two reasons. The first reason is because you need a new refrigerator, and the second reason is because we love you. Now, will you come with us to pick one out?"

"Okay, if you're sure. Are you really sure?"

Becky hugs me. "Very sure. Let's go find Dave and go pick something out for you."

By the time we get back to the house, things are pretty much in order. Furniture is in place, the kitchen is put together, and Alice is in one bathroom, while Judy is in the other, both unpacking boxes of towels and toiletries. I'm wondering if people have stopped to eat when I see the lunch sacks and the coolers of drinks. Susan and John Roach, from church, have brought two big coolers of soft drinks and another of bottled water. That they thought to include water somehow just hits me, and the tears start to flow. How will I ever pay all these people back? How?

Mostly the days are spent trying to adjust to this new normal. I scour the papers for want ads and do see an office manager job that I think I can do. I call, and after a brief conversation, get an appointment for an interview. Hope surges through me. Hope for a job, hope for an income, hope for medical insurance.

I take a psychological test after the interview, but I do explain that I have been a widow for two weeks so the results might be a little skewed at this sitting. I think the interviewer is somewhat impressed or amazed by my apparent calmness because she invites me back for a second interview before she even looks at the psychological test results. We set the appointment for the next week. I'm glad she doesn't see the inside of me—the fear, the pain, the uncertainty.

Despite the circumstances, it is wonderful to be back in our house, but it is not wonderful to have a swimming pool in the back yard that has not had the care that it needed. Apparently, either the pump or filter quit working sometime in the late spring while the tenants were here, and they didn't know what to do so they ignored it or they just ignored it because they did not care. Either way, the result is a giant cement hole in the back yard that is full of gruesome-looking water. Samuel has been diligently working on cleaning it but to no avail. I get gallons of chlorine, spending money we need for necessities, and we dump gallon after gallon into the murky water. Our eyes are watering, and I know if one of us got in the pool, whatever clothes on the body would be bleached white. I don't see much change in the water though, and I shout, "I'm just going to call someone to fill it in with cement! Not that I have the money for that because I don't have money for anything, much less this pool!"

"Go in the house, Mom. I'll take care of the pool. Something will work; I'll keep trying until it does." Samuel's response is gentle as he continues to brush the sides of the pool.

It does take a while, but within another week, the water is clear, and we can get back in the pool. This is important for Elizabeth especially because she loves swimming, and it gives her something to do on these long, hot days of July. I look at the water, formerly murky but now clear and inviting. How I wish that were my mind and my life—clear and inviting—but that is not to be. Not now. I can't help but wonder, will my life ever be like that again?

My eyes pop open, and my heart is racing. In my dream, the IRS has knocked on the door to tell me that my house is no longer mine. The IRS is seizing it as payment for the taxes that Dennis didn't pay six or seven years ago. This is what he was talking about when he met with the IRS about a month before he died. He told me I didn't need to worry, but I have to find out exactly what can happen. From the phone book,

I get a number for an attorney specializing in tax work and after breakfast, call for an appointment. He assures me that the IRS cannot seize my house, and, in fact, will not do anything without notifying me first. "You can't ignore this forever, Mrs. Curtis, but for right now, you can take this off your list of worries."

The day before my third and final job interview, the phone rings. "Hello?"

"Mrs. Curtis? This is Mr. Dominguez at Thomas Jefferson. Are you still interested in teaching for us?"

"Teaching at TJ? Yes, I am. Without a doubt."

"Okay, then, here's what I need you to do. Get your resume down to Personnel this afternoon, and you've got a job. Do you know where to go?"

"Yes, Sir, on Ross Avenue. That's all I need to do, take my resume down there and you've got a teaching job for me?"

"That's right. It won't be a reading position, but I'll have something for you. You've just got to take that paperwork down there today. Can you get there today?"

"Yes, I'll be there within the hour."

"Good, good. Now new teachers report next week, so come by here today or tomorrow, and I'll give you the schedule. Welcome back to Thomas Jefferson, Mrs. Curtis."

My mind is racing when I hang up the phone. In the three weeks since July 13th, I've gone from getting a teaching job, to losing a teaching job, to having a potential job somewhere else, and now to having a teaching job. I remember that I have a choice now because AIDS is no longer a factor. Is this what I want to do? Teach? The salary, $26,000, is about the same with the other job, but if I teach, I will have a schedule that resembles Drew and Elizabeth's, and that is important right now. Heading to the file drawer, I find the paperwork I need and head to 3700 Ross Avenue. Time will tell me if this is the right decision, but for now, I know I have a job, and that is what I need to know.

st Keep Breathing

Two days later as I think about a daily schedule, the first problem arises. How am I going to get Drew and Elizabeth to school? I have to be at school at 7:15 a.m. and classes start at 7:30 a.m. Drew and Elizabeth cannot get to school before 8:00, but even Samuel will already be in classes since he'll be with me at TJ. We have one neighbor who has children at Good Shepherd, so I call them. I don't believe it, but my schedule works perfectly with theirs. Mrs. Johnson is a nurse and works the afternoon/evening shift. She can take them in the morning if I can pick them up, which I can because I get out forty-five minutes before they do. *Thank You, God, for helping me not give up at each little obstacle.*

CHAPTER 17

Look to the Light

Before I know it, we have gotten through Elizabeth and Drew's August birthdays and school has started. I am teaching classes of students who are newcomers to our country, meaning they have very little knowledge of the English language. I have no idea what I am supposed to do, so I hang pictures of objects, we talk about vocabulary and try to find some commonalities between Spanish and English.

Towards the end of August, it is time for Kathryn to head back to Ohio and school. Her friend Ryan from her sophomore year has called, learned about Dennis, and will be there with a strong shoulder when she needs it. My heart breaks at the thought of her leaving us. Somehow having her here has helped me because we have all been together, but I know she is just the first to leave and slowly, they will all leave. I call in sick on the day she leaves. I call in sick the next day, too. Mrs. Mason, the Dean of Instruction, calls me during the afternoon of my second day at home. "Mrs. Curtis, how are you feeling?"

"Oh, a little better, thank you."

"Mrs. Curtis, I do understand what is happening, but it won't solve anything for you stay home. The only way for you to move forward is to come back to school and teach. Come back every day and let one day become another and another and another. You will be busy teaching, and you won't even notice how quickly the days go from one to the next. Today is Friday, so you've got the weekend to rest, and I'll expect to see you Monday. Okay?"

"Yes, Ma'am. Thank you for understanding. I will be there Monday."

Monday morning there is a note in my box to go see Mr. Dominguez during my planning period. Apparently, the reading teacher sent from the central office has walked off the job, and I can have the reading job if I want it. I don't really know any more about teaching reading than I do about teaching English to newcomers, but I welcome the change because I do like to read and maybe I'll do more of that in my new assignment. Right now I am numb to most everything around me. The students in my classes are nice kids, but I keep myself removed because I don't want to feel anything. I know I have to do something to get past this numbness because these kids that I am teaching deserve more than I am able to give right now.

One of the teachers at Good Shepherd tells me about a grief recovery group that will have a six-week session beginning in mid-September. This teacher lost her husband two years ago and found this program quite helpful. I call the church where it will be held, inquire about times and procedures, and enroll. I attend on Thursday nights for two hours, and Samuel stays at home with Drew and Elizabeth. No one has soccer practice that night so it works perfectly. There are twelve of us in the group, and the losses vary both in relationship and in time passed, but the common link is loss, and we are all grieving. We read, we write, we talk. This group helps me because I don't have to hide anything here. I don't cry, though. I'm scared that if I start, I might not stop.

Just as Mrs. Mason said, the days fold into one another and all of a sudden it is October. We have always carved several pumpkins for jack-o-lanterns, and I have always done some little decorating for Halloween. This year, I don't want to do anything. I'm exhausted when I get home every day, and the thought of decorating for Halloween is overwhelming. I look at Elizabeth, however, and know I have to do something. It's not her fault that she's only eight years old and has expectations beyond October 31 just being a date on the calendar.

One afternoon, we go to Michael's, an arts and crafts store, to find some Halloween decorations.

Elizabeth is excited; this is the sort of thing we used to do. As I walk up and down the aisles, nothing appeals to me, and it all is so expensive, way beyond my budget. Inside my head, I am screaming, *I hate this day! Whoever thought up pumpkins and witches and ghosts anyway? It is all so stupid!* Then I hear a little voice, "Mommy, can we get these little pumpkins? They're only five dollars, and two is all we need. We could put those little candles in them, and I know we have some of those, and we can use these next year, too."

I look at her. She is looking at me expectantly, but there is such sadness in her eyes. "Yes, Sweet Pea, these little jack-o-lanterns are perfect. Thank you for finding them. I think this is all we need because we'll get real pumpkins at the grocery to carve, don't you think? We can put these in the dining room on the mantle." We buy the ceramic pumpkins, and maybe both of us have a moment of feeling better.

November first is All Saints Day, and I receive notice from the church that a worship service will be held that evening, and Dennis' name will be called out along with the name of every member who has died this year. I know we have to go to this service. That day at school, Samuel's English teacher, Mrs. Young, brings me a copy of Samuel's journal page. She does not normally share their journal writing, but she is concerned about Samuel's well-being and feels she needs to share it with me. He writes, "November 1, 1995. Tomorrow is my birthday, but I will not turn seventeen without my father here to witness it. Last night I had to take my little sister and brother trick-or-treating. That's what my father always did before. I went to my girlfriend's after work, and we were studying when my mother called and asked me to take them because she was too tired. I know she wasn't really too tired. It just made her too sad. I did it and then went back to my girlfriend's.

Halloween didn't turn out like I thought it would, but it wasn't that bad."

Mrs. Young doesn't know how to take the statement, "I will not turn seventeen without my father here to witness it." I thank her and tell her I will handle it from here. When I ask Samuel about later, he just says, "All it means is that in a way, I'll always be sixteen, the age I was when Dad died."

That evening we go to the worship service at church. Well, Drew, Elizabeth, and I go. Samuel is working and will go to his girlfriend's after work. The service is beautiful—uplifting hymns, thought provoking words, hope-inspiring scripture—and then Blair begins calling out the names. Drew remains stoic, but Elizabeth can't take it. She is sobbing. I pull her to me and hold her tight. We get through all the names, the service comes to a close, and we leave. On the way to the car, Elizabeth looks up at me, "Mommy, don't ever make me come to something like that again." And there's my reminder again. They have lost their father, and how could I ever make up for that?

A few days after Samuel's birthday on the second of November, a student bursts into my classroom. "Mrs. Curtis, Ms. Allen says to come fast. It's Samuel." Ms. Allen, the school nurse, wants me because of Samuel?

"What's wrong? Who's going to watch my class?"

"She's getting someone, but she says to come now because he can't walk." I am almost running out of the door before he finishes his sentence.

When I get to the nurse's office, Samuel is lying on the bed. "Joan, Samuel's legs are giving him problems. They seem to be too weak to support him. You need to get him to the doctor, and preferably today."

Oh my word, what is wrong with him? *Please, God, let him be okay. Don't let it be a brain tumor or anything. I can't take anything happening to him.*

I am able to get him into the doctor right away. One of the coaches helps me get him to the car, and by the time we get to the doctor, he feels strong enough to walk with my support. After a battery of tests are run, the diagnosis is simple and, thankfully, not terminal. He is the .001 percent of people who have a side-effect to Lithium, the drug he's been taking to treat the bipolar depression. The doctor stops the Lithium immediately and gives me a prescription of an alternative drug. I don't even know how to describe what is going through me, except it feels like someone just blew breath back into me so I could resume my breathing. An alternative drug for which I'm grateful, but this one will cost more and that means another pull on an already strained budget.

Twenty-six thousand dollars does not go far when you are feeding a family of five, much less buy this kind of medication. Luckily, I am getting some social security, but I don't have much left over for anything extra. When I think about the Christmases that our children have experienced, I realize that I have to have a second job if I am even going to have a Christmas tree. I see a job posting for seasonal help at The Container Store in the classified ad section of the paper. I love The Container Store—you can find any kind of organizational container that you want there, and the sales staff is always so nice. I apply, interview, and get the job. I will begin in late November, work two weeknights, plus one day on the weekend, and continue through the end of January.

Kathryn comes home for Thanksgiving, and Mother insists we go to Longview. I'm not sure what is the right thing to do for the kids, but I do know that I cannot cook Thanksgiving dinner this year. Mother won't cook; we'll go out to eat, and she'll take care of making reservations. I don't know why this upsets the kids. It's one day. We drive down that morning and come back that evening. On the way home, Elizabeth remarks, "I didn't know you could get turkey and dressing in a restaurant. It was like we really had Thanksgiving dinner." Now I get it. My children have always had Thanksgiving dinner at home. They thought if we went out, we'd be eating hamburgers or Mexican food, not the traditional turkey and dressing. Yes, we need to communicate better.

Before I take Kathryn to the airport, I take a picture for our Christmas card. We have had a picture on every Christmas card since Kathryn's birth in 1974. I get home from the airport and get the camera to remove the film and take it to the drugstore, but when I open the camera, there is no film. No film, no picture. Shaking my head in frustration, I realize, how appropriate. Of course, our Christmas card would be different this year; everything is different now.

One Sunday in December, while working at The Container Store, it starts snowing. Light flakes float down and gently fall on the pavement. About 2:00 p.m. I grab my coat and run across the street to La Madeleine for lunch. I get the cream of mushroom soup, and as the warm liquid slides down my throat, I watch the snowflakes fall. *Your world is beautiful, God. I don't see the beauty much these days, but I see it right now, and it is overwhelming.* I can actually feel the movement as the smile covers my face.

Exams begin at school as we inch nearer to the break for Christmas. I am so ready to be home for two whole weeks. Grief is such an exhausting emotion that I find it difficult to have the energy for much outside of school, Container Store, soccer games, and basketball games. I haven't graded nearly enough papers, but I know I'll have time over the break to get them done. Kathryn will be home, so we'll all be together for a while. I'm anxious to hear about her friend, Ryan. Samuel has told me that Ryan has become more than a friend. Following the exams on the last day, I get my paperwork turned in and pack the papers to take home with me. Then it hits me. We are going to celebrate Christmas, and Dennis won't be there. He won't be there to shop on Christmas Eve like we always do. He won't be there to wrap a multitude of gifts in old-fashioned Santa paper at the last moment like we always do. He won't be there to breathe his magic into Christmas Eve and Christmas Day. He won't be there. I feel like a ten-ton boulder hits me right in the stomach and knocks me back into my chair. *Okay, God, if he won't be there, I won't go home. I'll just stay here.* I sit in silence, unable or unwilling to move, until I hear no more footsteps in the hall. Then I continue to sit. And sit. And sit. Finally, it is 4:00, and I have been alone since 1:00. Slowly, I rise, pick up my bag of papers, remind myself to just keep breathing and head home.

Early on the afternoon of Christmas Eve, I hear the doorbell. When I open the door, no one is there, but an envelope marked "Elizabeth" is taped to the corner of the porch rail. Elizabeth is right behind me so I hand it to her. Sliding her finger under the flap, she is excited to be getting a surprise. She pulls out The Gap gift card-holder, and her jaw drops when she looks at the card. "It is for a hundred dollars at The Gap!" she squeals.

I quickly look down the street but see nothing. There is no clue who did this, but I have my thoughts. I'm sure a few of the mothers at Good Shepherd did this for her and want no credit. They just love Elizabeth and want to show it somehow. Elizabeth is really excited and runs to show Kathryn because the two of them have plans to go shopping together after Christmas. I know I will never forget this day. While Elizabeth may not remember it, I will always know that this act let her believe that good things still happen. And for an eight-year-old who watched her father wither away to nothing, knowing that good things still happen is perhaps the most powerful knowledge to have.

Sometime in early January, I notice dark circles under Drew's eyes. He looks so tired, and I know I need to find out what the problem is, as if losing his father isn't enough of a problem. "I can't sleep, Momma, because it's almost Dad's birthday, and I just keep thinking about how sick he was last year. Remember? The only reason he even made an effort to get out of bed was because Elizabeth asked him to come open his presents. I just can't get that picture of him out of my mind, and it's keeping me from sleeping."

Dennis' birthday is, or am I supposed to say was, January 29, and I can see that this date is really troubling Drew. Several years ago during a Kennedy remembrance on November 22, Dennis had commented to me that he wanted to be remembered on his birthday and not on the day that he died. That memory helps me know what I need to do to help Drew.

On January 29, I take the day off and keep the kids home from school. We go to lunch at Dave & Buster's, a local restaurant with a game arcade. We had been frequent patrons there when Dennis was alive, and it was always a fun occasion. On this day, the kids play a few games, and we each share a good memory of their father. Certainly, this doesn't take the pain away, but for a few hours, we are intentional about celebrating Dennis' life instead of mourning the loss of it.

CHAPTER 18

Eyes Open to the Goodness

My job at The Container Store is coming to an end by mid-February, and I know I am going to miss this place. Although my reason for taking it was to have some money for Christmas gifts, the real benefits are that I've been able to spend some time each week in an adult world, and I've met Mel. Mel also works at The Container Store, and he and I have become fast friends. We laugh, we commiserate, we talk, we listen. I don't have to be any certain way with Mel because he takes me just as I am on that given day.

On one of the last days that I work, I see Mel talking to a couple about an over-the-door ironing board. That little ironing board has been a life saver for me these past few months because I can quickly iron Drew and Elizabeth's shirts each morning before school. I don't have the energy to plan much ahead, so I wash the clothes on the weekend, and each morning I grab a shirt for both of the kids, flip that ironing board down, press quickly, flip the board back up, and I'm done in less than five minutes. I know that in the grand scheme of things, this ironing board doesn't rate high on the list, but in my life right now, everything seems monumental, so if this little item seems to make one thing smaller in scope, it is high on the list in my world.

Having removed the red Container Store apron because I'm on my way to lunch, I stop by Mel and his customers. "If you are thinking about this product, I think it is one of the best conveniences in this store."

"Do you use one of the boards? You don't find it too small for some pieces of clothing?"

"To the contrary," I reply to the woman who has asked the question. "Because it is smaller, I can have it down and back up in less than ten minutes and have ironed shirts for my son and daughter. I don't have to spend a lot of time straightening the fabric on a big board. Believe me, this is one of the best things I've run across, and I use it every day before I go to work." I look at Mel, "You can have your customers back now."

"Thank you for your input," Mel responds and then winks.

As I am walking out of the door, I hear the gentleman tell Mel, "I don't know who she is, but you all ought to hire her for this store. She's a great saleswoman." Chuckling to myself, I feel a warm glow. Since I don't really know much about teaching reading and writing, I don't have much self-confidence in my everyday job of teaching, but at least this comment lets me know that I can do something well.

The job at The Container Store ends, Mel and I promise to keep in touch, and I return to my world of children and adolescents. Certainly, my students have made their ways into my heart even if I know I'm not their best teacher. I have this class of seniors, all of whom speak Spanish as their first language, and they all need to pass the state standardized test in reading or writing in order to graduate. There are only eight students in this class, and we really do have a good time together. For all the grammar rules, we use short texts containing grammatical errors. I sit on my desk with Starbursts in my hand. When a student reads the text, finds an error and explains why it is an error and how to correct it, I toss a Starburst in recognition. Even if the student is wrong, a Starburst goes flying through the air. I am rewarding risk, not correctness. Only if they take the risk to answer aloud can I help them move from misconceptions about English grammar.

By the end of the school year, six of the eight students have passed whatever state test they needed to pass. On their last day of school, I give them all a letter thanking them for everything they have given me this year. A reason to get up each morning, a reason to leave my house, a reason to smile because they have wanted to learn something from me, and I want them to know the difference that knowing them has made for me. As difficult as this year has been, they have given me so much more than I could possibly have imparted to them. These students have given me the knowledge that I am important, and as much as I hope I won't remember too much about this year of loss and adjustment, I know I will never forget them.

Mother gives me the money for us to go to Ohio for Kathryn's graduation from Miami. It's a fun weekend, and we meet Ryan's parents, too. Kathryn and Ryan are both moving to Texas. They will look for jobs, and I agree to let Ryan stay with us until they can save enough money for an apartment. I am so excited to have Kathryn home again, and she knows she has to live in Texas for the realization of her father being gone to really take hold. She also knows that both Elizabeth and I need her home for a while. For Mother's Day, Kathryn rounds all the kids up and makes them plant flowers in the beds by the pool. Ryan, Kathryn, and Samuel paint the exterior of the house. As they get involved in their tasks, I am wondering how I managed without them.

Needing to supplement my income, I apply to teach summer school and am accepted. I teach eighth graders who failed the state test in reading and/or math and are, therefore, required to attend summer school to go to the ninth grade. This involves a fairly set curriculum, and it's only in the morning four days a week, so Samuel will be able to stay with Drew and Elizabeth until I get home each afternoon following lunch.

The extra money coming in gives me the freedom to think a little past each paycheck, and I decide to have a party on the Fourth of July. I know the kids will all leave one day and have other commitments around holidays, so I cannot expect them to come home every Thanksgiving and every Christmas. But the Fourth of July—well, we live in a hot state, and I do have a swimming pool. I can expect them home for the celebration, so we will start it this summer, July 4, 1996. I am excited because this summer school money will allow me to have a celebration like we used to have.

The last week of summer school is the first week of July. I cash my paycheck so that I can physically take the cash for each bill and put it aside, and see exactly how much money I will have for the party. On Tuesday, I take $215.00 to school so that I can go buy all the food and supplies before I go home. The last bell rings, and I leave after my last student so that I can turn in my roll sheets for the day. When I get back to my room, I open the bottom desk drawer and see my open purse and no billfold. I run to the office to report the theft, and in walks one of the custodians. He has just found the contents of my billfold in one of the commodes in the boys' restroom. I now have a wet driver's license, a wet insurance card, a wet faculty ID, and no cash. All of my money is gone. *Please, God, what am I doing wrong? What am I not learning? What? I just don't understand why this happened? I don't know why You would let this happen. Why?*

The next morning one of the teachers brings me fifty dollars. She apologizes for the fact that there isn't more that she can share. I am speechless. She didn't steal my money, but here she is, apologizing that she can't replace it. *Okay, God. I know. You didn't take the money, but You did put this person here to offer me something of hers. I see. There is always more good than there is bad. I will always end up in the light. Always.*

About three months later, I can see that Drew and Elizabeth need a lift. I know I am about out of money, but I think a trip to Herrera's is something we all need. Herrera's was Dennis' favorite restaurant, and it is another place we frequented and had such fun. We would always get Laffy Taffy when we left, and Elizabeth would make up jokes like the ones inside the Laffy Taffy candies. No matter the answers given to the riddles, Mommy was always right and everyone else was always wrong. Yes, dinner at Herrera's would do us all good. Checking my resources, I have thirty-five dollars, milk, and bread. It's Tuesday, I get paid on Friday, and Samuel will be at work so it is just Drew, Elizabeth, and me. That means we can eat at Herrera's for fifteen dollars. We go, and we all leave full of warm enchiladas and good memories. As we walk through the parking lot, we each have a pepper-mint in our mouths and a Laffy Taffy in our hands. I am lost in memories.

Just before we get to the car, a woman approaches and speaks to me, "Excuse me, Ma'am, but can you spare any money? My husband just threw me out of the house, me and my boy, and we haven't eaten anything today. I just gotta get him somethin' to eat before I find someplace for us to stay the night. Can you help me? Please?"

I think of the twenty dollars in my purse. I think of the milk and bread at home. I think of the paycheck that is coming on Friday, just three days from now. I think of the fifty dollars that teacher gave me during summer school after my money was stolen. I want this woman to know that there are more good people in the world than there are bad. I open my purse and hand her my last twenty dollars.

CHAPTER 19

An Answer to a Prayer

I am finding the second year of teaching enthralling. I guess it isn't the teaching that is so enthralling but the students. They are eager to learn, and paramount for some of them, is the knowledge that education is the only way they will ever change their lives. I am becoming friends with teachers, and those that teach my content of reading and writing are ready to help me in any way that they can. Alice has put me in contact with one of the English teachers on her campus, and that teacher is sharing ideas and strategies and texts with me. I am still unsure of myself, but my students don't seem to care. They like being in my class, and they like coming in before and after school to talk.

Things at home are settling down, too. Samuel finally has a trustworthy car, and between school, work, and his girlfriend Amory, we rarely see him. Drew is holding his own at Good Shepherd and having fun playing soccer. He is finally on the Comets with Bradley, and that certainly soothes the wound from last year when he failed to make the team. Elizabeth is enjoying fourth grade, and even her third grade teacher has told me that she now sees a real smile on Elizabeth's face at school. Kathryn and Ryan are engaged, gainfully employed, and sharing an apartment. We get together at least once a week and have dinner. William has received a scholarship, so he is back in school at the University of Texas at Dallas and tending bar at night to support himself.

It seems I have made a successful transition from married stay-at-home mom to single-parent teacher. I like what I do. I have made a place for myself at Thomas Jefferson. I've helped chaperone a field trip of five days in New York

City. I was even interviewed on the news about the reading program that we use, and I've found a reading conference to attend in San Antonio, made reservations, and received district funds to attend. The view from the outside is that we are going through all the right motions, and the Curtis family is doing great. We are on our way.

But that's the view from the outside. From the inside, we are only going through the motions. I keep thinking this is all just temporary, that I'm on a trip somewhere, and, eventually, it's going to end. I'll go home, Dennis will be there, and we'll resume the life we had before the AIDS diagnosis in March of 1994. My children gave me a sterling silver AIDS bracelet that is called "Until There's a Cure." I wear it every day, but it is simply an adornment for my arm. I'm not connected to it, not in any real way. Maybe it is too much for me to absorb. Dennis was infected with HIV for thirteen years, and I'm not infected? How in the world could that have happened? How?

I'm sitting in the auditorium at Thomas Jefferson contemplating all these thoughts. Exciting events are on the horizon—Kathryn and Ryan are getting married in June, the reading conference in San Antonio in July. Why do I not *feel* more excitement?

Okay, God, I need Your help here. I survived. I didn't die; I'm not infected; I'm here, still breathing. I don't know why I'm not infected, but You must have some other purpose for me. So I've survived, but I've got to learn how to embrace life again. I don't know how to be a better mother. I don't know how to be a better friend. I'm not a wife anymore. I just know I have to do something different so I can really live life. Not just survive, but embrace life and be happy, truly happy, again. I've got to do this for me, and I've got to do this for my children, to show them that is what you do when life beats you down. So what do I do, God? What do I do to take back my life?

All of a sudden I know what I need to do. My students deserve the most informed teacher that

I can be, so that means I need to go back to school. I got an undergraduate degree twenty-two years ago in speech pathology. Now I need to learn about reading because something tells me it's more than these packets of worksheets I'm distributing every day. I understand caring; now I need to know about reading. It's funny, but I can feel the excitement welling up inside me. It's small, but it's there.

CHAPTER 20

Just Keep Breathing

Following an absolutely beautiful wedding where Kathryn is given away in marriage by her brothers, I get serious about registering for school. I inquire about requirements at the University of Texas at Dallas, Texas Woman's University, and East Texas State University. Any of these schools would be within commuting distance. Because I had taken a few graduate courses in the early eighties, I have already taken the Graduate Record Examination, so I inquire about the necessity of obtaining those records. Two of the schools tell me that I will have to take the GRE again because my scores on the previous exam are outdated. However, Texas Woman's University has a different approach. One time with the GRE is enough if I scored high enough, and I did. The other deciding factor is that TWU offers a Master of Arts in Secondary Reading, and because that is a critical need area in Dallas ISD, the school district will reimburse me for books and tuition. Mother will help me by advancing the money for the first semester, and I will use the reimbursement from the district for subsequent semesters. I decide to enroll at Texas Woman's University in Denton, Texas. I meet with an advisor and find a course on Monday evening, which meets at Presbyterian Hospital in Dallas. This is meant to be—no one has soccer on Monday, and the class meets in Dallas. I know I am going in the right direction.

Elizabeth rides with me to Denton to pay the fees for the first semester. "Sweet Pea, I know you don't like the idea of me being gone at night, but it is only one night each week. You'll be okay."

"I know, Mommy. I just wish you didn't go."

"I'm sure you can't really understand this right now, Sweet Pea, but I am doing this as much for you as I am for me."

"What do you mean, for me? How is your going to school going to help me, Mommy?"

"Well, you're ten years old now, right? That means in eight years, you will be eighteen and ready for college. I'm going to school now so I can start building a life for myself, so when you're eighteen and ready for college, you'll know you can go anywhere you want to go instead of thinking that you have to stay close to home since your mother will be alone after you leave. That's how I'm doing this for you, my love."

"I do understand that, Mommy, but I'll miss you when you're at school."

It's hard for me to believe how easy this has all been, and now the one complication is that Drew has a soccer tournament in Arlington on the first Monday of class because that Monday is Labor Day. Our friends the Nappers will bring him home, so that complication quickly dissipates. A week before class is to begin, I get a phone call that the class has been cancelled, but there is one other class on Monday night if I would like to switch to that one. It is Assessment of Reading and is required for my degree, so I agree to enroll there. The one problem is that it meets on campus in Denton, but I'll just make that work.

Labor Day weekend arrives, and we are in Arlington most of the time watching Drew play soccer. On Monday, Kathryn and Ryan come over to stay with Elizabeth, and Drew and I go to the tournament. Before I know it, it is time to leave and head to class. I've carefully mapped out the best way to get from Arlington to Denton, and I choke back tears as I wish Drew good luck.

It seems to take forever to get to I-35, the road to Denton, but I'm finally there and headed north. I am so jittery, wondering how I'll make this all work. I haven't been to school in over fifteen years, and when I went back then, at least I knew something about the field I was studying. Now I know nothing about what I'm about to study. For a moment I laugh about the irony in the fact that I'm teaching in a field about which I feel I know nothing. By the time I cross Lewisville Lake and am about twenty minutes from campus, I have to pull off the road for a minute. The tears burn my cheeks as they fall. I have no idea what I'm doing or how I'm going to do it. I remember Dave's words. Just keep breathing, Joan. Just keep breathing. I wipe the tears away, put the car in drive, and pull back onto the freeway.

CHAPTER 21

A New Beginning

There are about eighteen people in this class, and the teacher is dressed in a suit—professional. I take a seat in the middle of the right row of desks, not too far from the door. I sit a little on the edge, maybe so I can bolt out the door if I feel the need. Looking around, I see a wide range of people—men, women, both older and younger than me, and not just Anglo faces. For some reason, these faces put me at ease because I was worried I would be in a class of twenty-four year olds.

Ms. Wickstrom, Carol Wickstrom the instructor, begins talking. She's a doctoral student at TWU, and this is her first graduate class to teach. She taught public school for over twenty years and every elementary grade except fourth grade.

As she goes through the syllabus, she fully explains each assignment. Right now it all seems overwhelming to me, but I'll try to take it just one assignment at a time, just the way I'm living life right now.

Now we're taking turns introducing ourselves. We have to say our names, what we do and if teaching now, what and where, and how did we get into teaching. Do I say that I'm a widow? I kind of like thinking I'm starting new, with a clean slate, and no one needs to know that I'm a widow. But then, that is why I got into teaching. If Dennis had not died, I would be at home with my kids right now. There's Mark, Lorenda, now it's my turn, and I don't know what to say. "Uh, I'm Joan Curtis. I teach in Dallas, ninth grade reading at Thomas Jefferson High School. I've only been teaching for two years; this is my third. I, uh, I started teaching because my husband died two years ago, and my children wanted to keep eating." I did it, and I'm okay. I think I can do this. I think I can.

I really enjoy going to class each week. It is difficult for Elizabeth, but I call her every week during the break, so that helps some. I have to keep reminding myself that this is for both of us, and it's true. I have to build a life for myself; that is a non-negotiable.

When we get our first assignments back, I am thrilled to see that I've gotten fifteen out of fifteen points. And what I really like is that Ms. Wickstrom doesn't just put "15/15" on the paper, she writes comments in different places. She asks questions; she connects what I've said to some text or idea; she affirms my thinking with, "Yes, and … You're on the right track." She even does this during our discussions. Building on what we say, she adds to it or takes it to a question we don't try to answer; we just ponder. I'm getting a little braver about speaking because I know she won't humiliate or belittle me. I'm beginning to feel like I know something of value.

During the break about mid-semester, I approach Ms. Wickstrom to ask her a question. She has told us that her father died when she was just twelve. She's erasing the board, and I'm a little unsure how to ask this question. "Ms. Wickstrom, I know your father died when you were just twelve. That's how old my youngest son was when my husband died. I want to help my children, but I don't have any idea what they're going through because I didn't lose a parent until I was thirty-four years old. Sometime, would you talk to me about how you learned to deal with your father's death, so I can help my children?"

Ms. Wickstrom slowly turns back to the board and then turns toward me. She has tears in her eyes, but a slightly amused tone as she replies, "I'll be glad to help you once I deal with my father's death for myself. And, Joan, please call me Carol. You're making me feel really old by calling me Ms. Wickstrom all the time."

By the last night of class, I know I don't want it to end. I really enjoy the time each Monday, and those three hours are among the fastest in the week. Carol has such a wonderful sense of humor, and we laugh so much in class. I have borrowed some books from Carol, so I decide I won't take them back tonight. That way, I can contact her in the spring, and we can set a time to meet, and I can return the books. She is the first person to treat me as an independent woman, and I don't want to lose that yet.

During the break, Carol asks me to come by her office before I go home. I panic. Did I not turn an assignment in? Is she mad because I was late to class tonight even though I called and explained why I'd be late? I feel silly. I'm forty-seven years old, and I feel like I've been called to the principal's office.

At the close of class, I go downstairs to Carol's office. "Did you want to see me?"

"Yes, Joan. You know, you just seem like someone I'd like to get to know, so I didn't want you to leave tonight until we've scheduled a time to have lunch."

I am almost speechless. "Okay, I'll come up here for lunch if you'll promise to come to Dallas later and have dinner and meet my children." Because she is leaving right after Christmas to go skiing and Elizabeth and I are going to Ohio, we make arrangements to have lunch on December 23. She gives me directions to her apartment.

On the way home from school that night, I call Kathryn to tell her that Carol wants to have lunch with me. I am in tears because I am excited that someone wants to know me. Dennis was such a likeable person. He was warm and could carry on a conversation with anyone because he had a way of getting people to talk about themselves. I always thought he was the one people were attracted to, and I was the quiet one, unnoticed, standing by his side.

This semester has done wonders for me. My identity as an adult has been as a wife and a mother. I have incredible friendships, but I have still identified myself through Dennis and my children. I'm not a wife anymore, and my children will grow up and leave me—three of them already have left. This semester, I've been treated as Joan, an independent woman and teacher and student. I've learned how to help my students by assessing where they are now, and I've done well. And now, someone even wants to know me, just me. This feels like an opportunity to reinvent myself. Whom do I want to be? Even now I know I don't really want to reinvent myself, but I do want to learn to live so that my children know they are not responsible for my happiness. I'm learning to see school as a way to my independence, and a way to rebuild my life. I make my next decision. On New Year's Day, January 1, 1998, I am going to take off my wedding ring.

CHAPTER 22

A Long Way Travelled

I look out at all the people here for graduation. My stomach is in such a twitter. I see everyone, well, everyone who lives close enough to come. My sweet granddaughter, Alyssa, is almost a year old now. Kathryn had her the previous Fourth of July, 2000, and you can see a difference in our family since her birth. She brought such a confirmation of life to us all. Samuel is not here because the Air Force has him in Okinawa. He, too, has married and has a five-year-old stepdaughter now. We never see Samantha as a step-anything. From the beginning, she was part of our family. I do see Kathryn and Ryan, Drew, Elizabeth, and William. This year, this month, May 2001, is momentous. I am receiving my Master of Arts this morning.

William will receive his Master in Finance next week. Drew graduates from high school in two weeks, and Elizabeth graduates from Good Shepherd at the end of the month. Alyssa will have her fill of commencement ceremonies by the end of the month, I'm sure.

As I continue to look around the coliseum, I can't stop smiling, thinking about how far we've come. I am more than halfway through paying the IRS debt that Dennis left from our taxes in 1988. I had tried to put that out of my mind, but about three years after his death, the debt loomed in my nightmares. After consulting with an attorney and being advised to file bankruptcy, I did that and then filed an innocent spouse case since I didn't know about the debt. The debt he left had climbed to over eighty-thousand dollars, but I won the case so my debt was reduced to a little over eight thousand, and that will be paid in just two years.

I hear my name called, and as I move forward to accept my diploma, I see Carol, Claudia,

Veriena, and Carol C. I have met these women while attending TWU, and they have all encouraged me to pursue my doctoral degree. Working hard during my time here has paid off both personally and professionally. I developed a reading program for teen-aged mothers that teaches them about reading to their children. My circle of friends is wider because I see Carol, Claudia, Veriena, and Carol C. as both colleagues and friends, and they are a blessing in my life.

I accept my diploma, as chills run up and down my spine. It's difficult to imagine that any graduation could mean as much as this one. I hear the clapping, and it sounds thunderous. I'm sure it really isn't, but I feel like I am walking on air. It's funny to think I didn't even go to my undergraduate ceremony because I took that degree for granted. But this one, this Masters degree, is different. Remembering where I was just six years ago, I take a deep breath and move on to retake my seat.

Outside, after the ceremony, we take pictures. Kathryn has invited everyone over for a celebration lunch, so after pictures, we head east to Allen for one of those occasions when you can feel the joy in the room. The excitement is written all over Judy's face. She is proud of her big sister and that pride is evident as she recounts her story from the morning. "I was talking to one of my store managers early this morning, and he said he was going to a graduation today, too, and I told him that my big sister was getting her masters. He said his brother was also getting a masters, but I told him that he didn't understand about my sister. 'My sister,' I said, 'my sister was widowed and left bankrupt six years ago. She had to file bankruptcy and win an innocent spouse case with the IRS to save her house, and she teaches in DISD.'"

We're all laughing. Judy puts my teaching in Dallas in the same category as Dennis dying and the whole bankruptcy IRS incident. My sister doesn't understand I don't teach for the administrators in this district; I teach for my students, so the district does not matter. I love my job and know that my students have given me a reason to get out of bed every day. Teaching has given me a purpose, and I know I've made a difference for a lot of the kids I've taught. What a great day this has been! Joan Scott Curtis, M.A.—it has a nice ring to it.

We get through all the graduations, and summer brings a more relaxed pace. I almost feel at a loss because for the first summer in a long time, I'm not taking any classes. One night in early July, I am lying awake waiting for Drew to come home. He's been staying out too late too often, and I think I've reached the end of my rope. In the morning, I catch him before he goes to work. "Drew, this isn't going to work. You've stayed out all night one time too many. Not only do I not understand how you can let me worry that something has happened, I don't want Elizabeth to think this is acceptable behavior. Like it or not, you are an older sibling, and she learns from you. Here's your choice. If you live here, you've got to live by the rules, and if you don't want to live by my rules, you can live somewhere else." I know Drew doesn't have the money to live somewhere else, so I have no doubt that he'll agree to live by the rules. "You do understand what I'm saying, right?"

"Yes, and I haven't meant to make you worry, so I'm sorry about that. I have to go to work now, so we'll talk when I get home. Okay?"

"That works, Honey. I'll see you later." I knew Drew didn't really want to worry me. He's had a rough time during these teenage years. By ninth grade he had really descended into intense grief and had become dangerously depressed. He had felt that only Samuel could understand what he was feeling, so with my heart breaking, I let my fifteen-year-old son go to South Carolina to live with his twenty-year-old brother. Samuel had moved to South Carolina two years after he graduated from high school as a way of distancing himself from the painful memories that Dallas held for him. While living there, he decided to join the Air Force as a way to afford college. Drew went with the intention of staying through high school. While he was gone, I developed a habit of listening to the song from *Les Miserables*, "God on high, hear my prayer . . . he's a boy . . . bring him home." By December Drew was ready to come home, so after Christmas Elizabeth and I drove to South Carolina to get him. He enrolled at TJ and graduated in three years.

When Drew came home from work that afternoon, he walked right into the kitchen. "Momma, I found a place to live so is it okay if I get my stuff tomorrow? I'm too tired now."

"You found a place to live?"

"Yeah, there's this girl that works at Ball's with me, and she has a roommate, and they said I could stay with them until I'm eighteen and can sign a lease myself."

"You mean you're really going to move out? Where do they live?" My heart is sinking. I never thought it would turn out like this.

"Yeah, it's probably the best thing to do. They just live down the street in the cul-de-sac, in back of that pink brick house. There's an apartment over the garage."

Now this strikes me as funny. Drew is moving out, but he's just moving down the street. Okay, this isn't what I wanted, but here we are so this will have to work, too. Maybe Drew will figure things out for himself because, really, that is what everyone has to do. I can't do it for him, and he can't live here continuing to do as he pleases. The next afternoon, I watch him gather his clothes, and he is gone. My wish for him is that he finds his way soon. I've done what I can for him, but it is now up to him. Knowing this, my heart still breaks. Joan, keep breathing. Just keep breathing.

For the first time in her life, Elizabeth begins the school year at a Dallas public school. She isn't going to TJ with me, but to Hillcrest, one of the other high schools in North Dallas. She isn't happy. In fact, in her words, I am ruining her life. I can't afford Ursaline or the Episcopal School of Dallas where all her friends from Good Shepherd are going, but I do think she will eventually like Hillcrest. It doesn't take long before she is at home there. I think I've done something right, after all.

One Sunday evening in October, I answer the phone. "May I speak to Joan Curtis, please?"

"This is she."

"Joan, this is Jackie Peck from the College Reading Association. I am so excited to tell you that you have won our Outstanding Master's Research Award for 2001."

"What? I've won the CRA award?" I can't believe this. I knew Cathy, my thesis chair, had submitted my thesis, but I won? I really won?

"Yes, Joan, you won. I am so excited. When I read the title of your thesis, "Moving Adolescent Mothers toward the Path of Educated Independence," I was hoping that it would win. This is the J. Estill Alexander Award for Future Leaders in

Literacy Education, and you have won. You will be able to come to the conference this year, won't you? We present our awards at a breakfast at the conference, and we want to you make a brief presentation about your research. Very brief, just a few minutes."

"Yes, I hope I can come. I will let you know. And thank you, Dr. Peck, thank you for calling. Bye."

"I do hope you can come. I want to meet you and talk to you. Congratulations, Joan. Job well done. Bye now."

I hang up the phone in shock and call Kathryn. "Guess what? My thesis won the College Reading Association award for master's research!" I'm really crying now.

"Mom, I can't understand you. Try to calm down and tell me again. You are okay, right?"

"Uh huh," and I pause to get myself under control. "Dr. Peck from Ohio just called, and I won the College Reading Association award for master's research."

"Wow! Mom, that is great. I am so proud of you."

"Can you believe it?"

"Yes, Mom, I can. You have worked so hard, and you deserve this recognition. Congratulations, Mom. I love you."

Carol comes home a little later. Carol moved in when she was finishing her dissertation and needed a place to stay without a year's lease. It has worked for me to have an adult in the house and have a little more money from the rent she has paid. It has worked for her to have a house. She got a job at the University of North Texas, and we've become good friends, so she has stayed. "Hey! You won't believe this, but Jackie Peck from Ohio called. I won the CRA award for most outstanding master's research. They'll present it at the conference. I'm just not sure I can afford to go."

"That is wonderful! Wonderful! Okay, the conference. I've got enough airline miles for a ticket because you have to go, and I have a room reserved already so that's no problem. This is so exciting! Have you called Cathy?"

"No, I need to absorb it first. Are you sure about the miles? Are you going to the conference?"

"Yes, I'm going, that's I why reserved a hotel room, and you're going, too. This is just so exciting."

About three weeks later we are in Florida at the conference. My name is announced at breakfast on Saturday, along with the dissertation winner. There is a brief presentation after breakfast, giving us both an opportunity to talk about our research. Just a few people come, but they ask good questions, and I can tell they are really interested. One of the professors asks if I will continue in this area of adolescent mothers and literacy for my dissertation. She has just assumed that I'm going on for a doctoral degree. This feels good. Somehow in the last six years, I have moved from pitiful widow to professional educator. I am reminded of a comment that Dennis made years ago. "Ya' know, Scott, you are the smart one. Why don't I stay home with the kids, and you go to work? You know you would be really successful at whatever you chose." I chuckle to myself. That was my husband, always a step ahead of his time. I glance up and smile. I know he's proud of me.

CHAPTER 23

Faith in the Future

In August of 2004, Elizabeth begins her senior year at Hillcrest, and I begin my last year at Thomas Jefferson. I made the decision two years prior that when Elizabeth graduated, I would quit my job, sell our house, and go to school fulltime so that I could finish my doctoral degree. Standing in my classroom early on the first day of school, I do not want to be here. It isn't that I don't want to teach, but I am ready to see where I go when I finish my Ph.D. And it's not that I want to rush Elizabeth's senior year, but I am tired and ready to move on with my life. For all the wonderful things that have happened since Dennis died, it has not been easy to be a single parent, and something inside of me is anxious to look at Elizabeth at graduation and say *we did it.*

The halls are filling up with students searching for classes so I walk out of my classroom to answer questions and help people find their way. Looking down the hall, I can't believe my eyes, but there's Carmen, and she looks really scared. Eons ago during one of our good years, Carmen worked for me, cleaning our house. I haven't seen her in about fourteen years, but I know that it is her. She's standing right behind a young man with Down Syndrome, and she has her hand on his shoulder. Oh my word! She's with Enrique, her son. I will never forget finding her on the floor of our bathroom in tears because it was Enrique's second birthday, and he couldn't walk yet. Her husband had said they could not celebrate his birthday until Enrique walked. Well, Enrique's walking now, and he looks a little frightened, too.

Making my way through the crowd of students, I call her name. She instantly recognizes me, and when I finally get to her, we genuinely hug each other. "Carmen, how are you? This is Enrique, right?" I gently take Enrique's hand in mine, "Hello, Enrique, I am Mrs. Curtis. Welcome to TJ."

"Oh, Mrs. Curtis, I am so glad to see you. Enrique has been at E.D. Walker Middle School for the past several years because that was the school where they had all the kids in special education. But this year, they said all the kids had to go to their home school. Look at all these kids, Mrs. Curtis. I'm scared. I'm scared for Enrique because he'll get lost in them." There are now tears running down her cheeks.

"It's okay, Carmen; it's okay." I let go of Enrique's hand and take her face in my hands. "Carmen, I am here, and I won't let anything happen to Enrique." Now I know why I'm still at TJ for this last year. "Let's go to the office and find out where Enrique needs to go." I take Carmen with one hand and Enrique with the other hand,

and we make our way through the crowd of students headed to the office.

We're in luck. Enrique's classroom is right down the hall from mine on the first hall. Carmen explains to his teacher that she will pick up her daughter first each day, so sometimes she might be a few minutes late. Mrs. Sampson responds, "That might be a problem because we will have to take the students who ride the bus around to the cafeteria because that is where their bus will come. On the days that you're late, you will need to come around and pick Enrique up in the back."

"Why can't Enrique come to my room when you take the other students to the bus? That way, Carmen knows she always gets him at the same place, no matter the time. Will that work?" My classroom is the first room on the hall which means all Carmen would need to do is come through the front door, and he'd be right there with me.

I can see the relief on Carmen's face. I tell her to stop by my classroom when she finishes talking with Mrs. Sampson, and I head back to my class. Not only is Carmen relieved, but I am relieved, too. I am now glad I'm still at TJ. This is going to be a good year.

One morning after class, one of my students, José, lags behind. "Miss, have you ever wanted to kill yourself?"

"No, José, why would you ask that?"

"Because no one likes me, Miss, and high school is hard when no one likes you." José is a quirky kind of kid, one with some learning difficulties, but I don't have a student who tries any harder than he does.

"Well, I know that is not true, that no one likes you, because I like you. What can I do to help you?"

"I don't guess you'd want to eat with me in the cafeteria, would you, Miss? No one sits with me there." Why doesn't he just stab me in my heart? School buses and school cafeterias are the most difficult channels to navigate when you're a bit different.

I eat lunch alone in my room every day and relish this time to myself, but I know I have to do something different now. "José, I eat lunch in my room, and I would love it if you brought your lunch down here to eat with me each day."

"Can I do that, Miss? Will they let me leave the cafeteria with my tray and come to your room?"

"Yes, José, they will because I am going down to the cafeteria right now and talk to the assistant principal who sits at the cafeteria door and tell him that you have my permission to bring your tray to my room. In fact, I'll meet you there today at C-lunch. You do have C-lunch, don't you?"

"Yes, Miss, I do. Thank you, Miss. Thank you." José heads to his next class, and I make plans to meet him at the cafeteria at 1:00.

When I explain the situation to Mr. Dupree, the assistant principal, he understands completely. José begins eating lunch with me that day, and before I know it, other students I teach have heard and come to join us. They, too, feel on the outside of things. By November, the lunch group has grown to eight students and because José was the first one, he has taken a leadership role, and the other students don't mind at all. This lunch gang has become more than I ever envisioned.

Most Friday nights in the fall, I go to football games to watch Elizabeth's team since she is a cheerleader. It's fun to see the place she has made for herself at this school, and she's begun dating a really nice young man. Ironically, his mother was the first person I met on the day I went to look at the school. During one of the last games, I am watching her cheer and suddenly remember that afternoon when Dennis, shortly before his death, sat down to write each of the kids a last letter. When I got home later and asked him if he had written them, he had simply said, "No, because I started with Elizabeth and realized I'm going to miss everything because she's so little now." My eyes fill with tears as I watch her jump into the air. Yes, Dennis, you were right. You are missing everything.

Before I know it, it is Thanksgiving and thoughts turn to Christmas plans. Because this will be our last Christmas in this house, I want to have everyone here. In addition to my children and grandchildren, I invite Mother, Judy and Marshall and Bryan, Alice, Becky and Dave, and Ryan's parents, Linda and Dave. Mother calls my brother Arthur and tells him that he and his partner, Dan, need to come because it is an important time for me. They agree. Samuel and Stacy and their three children, Samantha, Dylan, and Austin are stationed in Alaska, so it is too far for them to come. All the other kids come, though. I really want everyone to sit at the same table, so we put two card tables at the end of the dining table and then add the entry hall table at the end. There are twenty-four of us, and the table stretches into the entry hall. What a magnificent day it is! One I will never forget. The laughter, the conversation, the food I've cooked every Christmas since I married in 1972. A toast to the years in this house, and we spend the next few hours eating, talking, remembering, laughing. I look at the people seated around these tables and know what a blessed life I have had. *Thank You, God, for these people. They have made my life so rich.*

January and February seem to evaporate, and March includes a trip to Austin for Elizabeth and me, and then it is gone, too. In April Elizabeth is notified by the financial aid department that she is in the running for a scholarship to the University of Texas at Austin. She responds with the requested confirmation that she plans to attend UT and then goes about requesting the recommendation letters from her teachers. Once she passes through that round, she passes through the phone interview, and then goes for a face-to-face interview. Next, the waiting begins.

After exams one afternoon, I am boxing more of my books when Elizabeth flies into my classroom. "I got it, Mom! I got it! A full scholarship covering everything!" I run to her and wrap her in my arms. We're both crying with excitement. This Terry scholarship is funded by a couple who made their money in oil and never had children. They set up this fund for educating students at four Texas schools in order to give back to the state that had richly rewarded them. It is not only money for tuition, books, room and board, but also extra living money in order for students to focus on studies and not work. And Elizabeth is one of the recipients. Wow!

On the last day of exams, one of my students asks me if I can take her home because her mother is not feeling well. "Of course, Mathilde, I will be happy to take you home after I take care of a few things in the office. Is it okay if we go in about thirty minutes?"

"No problem, Miss. I'll just wait in here."

Mathilde gives me directions to her house, and we are in her driveway within fifteen minutes of leaving the school. "Mi madre wants to meet you, Miss, because I've talked a lot about you. Will you come in and meet her?"

"Are you sure, Mathilde? Maybe she would rather not meet me right now since she isn't feeling well."

"No, Miss, it's okay. She told me to bring you in when we got here."

We get out of the car, and I follow her into her house. "Surprise!" shout about twenty-five of my students in the living room. Balloons and banners decorate the walls. "We love you, Mrs. Curtis" "Thank you, Mrs. Curtis, for helping make our lives different." "Good-bye, Mrs. Curtis, don't forget us." Nachos, enchiladas, tamales, chips and salsa, guacamole are in abundance on the table. How in the world did they pull this off? About an hour later, I am headed home, heart and stomach overflowing. What a day!

On my last day at TJ, I load the last box of books into my car. Walking down to the library to tell Cholly, my colleague and friend, good-bye, I decide to walk around the school one last time. In so many ways, this place saved me. My students gave me a reason to get out of bed and have some purpose in my life. Certainly, I had to keep going for my own children, but now I know that I am called to teach, and my students have taught me that. The friends and colleagues I've made in the ten years I've taught here have reminded me over and over to just keep breathing when I have been discouraged.

With that last thought, a memory rushes over me. In 1995, Linda, at the Virginia law office, asked me if I was okay when she realized that Dennis really was terminally ill. I told her no but to give me ten years and I would be okay. And here I am ten years later. Kathryn, Samuel,

Drew, and William are grown and settled into their own lives. Elizabeth has a full scholarship and will be leaving for school in two months. I have paid off the IRS and am completely out of debt. I have obtained a Masters degree and have resigned my teaching job here to go to school fulltime and finish my doctoral degree. Here I am exactly ten years later, and I am definitely okay. I head back to my classroom, pick up my purse, and walk out the door.

Afterword

On the eighth day of the eighth month in the year 2008, I was hooded with my Ph.D. in reading education. Despite being sick with hepatitis contracted as a side-effect to an antibiotic, the day was one I will never forget. My children, except for Samuel who was still in Alaska, were there, along with my three granddaughters. Mother, my sister Judy and her husband Marshall were there, too. My brother, Arthur, had died the previous March, and it is significant that I was able to get back to writing a dissertation after his death. When my name was called, I could hear Kiera, at two-years-old, the youngest of Kathryn's daughters, yell, "Go Mimi!" Tears filled my eyes. I knew my children were proud of me, but I wanted my grandchildren to remember me as someone who never let adversity stop me. I wanted all seven of my grandchildren to say, "That's our grandmother."

My children are leading happy productive lives although I know that the loss of their father has influenced their behaviors and decisions. In trying to understand their loss, I read several books concerning children and loss. One of the pieces of information I read stated that young children have two beliefs shattered when they lose a parent. As children, we believe that our parents are invincible and that they can solve anything. Of course, we eventually outgrow both of those beliefs. But for young children who lose a parent, they don't have the chance to outgrow them, and that changes the way these children see the world. I worried for a long time about this and kept trying to make up for their loss. I know that nothing can make up for a loss, but that didn't stop me from trying for too long. It wasn't that I finally realized that it was fruitless effort; it was that I finally accepted the fact that my children endured a terrible loss, and they would have to come to terms with that loss themselves.

After graduating from Miami of Ohio, Kathryn moved back to Dallas because she knew her little sister, Elizabeth. and I both needed her close. Kathryn worked in the financial realm until she had Alyssa, and now she and Ryan have three darling girls. Kathryn's life is much like mine was before her father died, busy with the activities of her girls and actively volunteering at their schools. Having had me at home for her entire childhood and adolescence, it was, perhaps the most difficult for Kathryn to adjust to me as an independent professional woman. Kathryn has always been the kind of person who could confront problems but only if she knew about them. Throughout Dennis' illness, I was withholding information from her, and the aftermath of that secrecy was a formidable force between us. But with time and much conversation, we have forgiven each other, and she is as proud of my accomplishments, as I am proud of hers.

Samuel really left home right after his father died. He was only sixteen and still in high school, so he still lived at home, but he spent the majority of his time divided between school, work, and his girlfriend's house. The year after he graduated from high school, he moved to South Carolina with his girlfriend, burying deeply the painful memories from home. Samuel joined the Air Force in 1999 and married his girlfriend. They divorced just a few months later while they were overseas. Samuel remained overseas, met his current wife online, and married her while he was stationed in Okinawa. They now have four beautiful children, three boys and a girl, and he has gotten an undergraduate degree in business education while serving his country and living in four different locations. He recently told me that it was time to face his loss because as painful as it is to face the past, it is exhausting to continue to run from it.

Drew had perhaps the most difficult journey just growing up because the grief hit hard when he was in middle school and stayed with him throughout his adolescence. He had to travel the hard road of addiction, but he found his way. When he studied abroad while a student at Texas Tech, he had an epiphany and knew he was on the road that led out of grief and into joy and reconciliation. After graduating from Texas Tech and working at Fidelity Investments for seven months, he called to tell me that he would never get job satisfaction from the corporate world and felt he was called to be a teacher. He quit his job nine months later and put himself through graduate school receiving a degree in curriculum and instruction. He and Amanda married two years ago in Ireland, and Drew began his teaching career this fall. Although he struggled through years of grief, he confronted his demons and runs no more. He and I can talk openly about our loss, how we each had a different loss, and how we've each chosen a career that matters for our lives and that helps give purpose to our experiences.

The Christmas following Dennis' death, I discovered about five hundred slips of paper buried in Elizabeth's closet. She had written either *Daddy* or *Dennis* on each piece of paper. That same year, her third grade class drew pictures of their families for Open House, and Elizabeth asked if she could put her daddy in the picture. Thankfully, her teacher had told Elizabeth that she could because her daddy would always be part of her family. Her teacher assured me all year that Elizabeth was doing well. However, when Elizabeth got to the fourth grade, this same teacher began to see what had been missing the previous year. Now she could see the smile in Elizabeth's eyes that had not been there before. It was during this fourth grade year that my youngest commented to me, "Life is getting good again, isn't it, Mommy?"

While Kathryn had a stay-at-home-mother, Elizabeth grew up with a working mother, and

this contributed to the independent woman she
has become. It was not an easy path for either
of us. She wanted the mother Kathryn had, and
I wanted to build the foundation for a life after
she left home. Unfortunately, I had to build the
foundation while she was still at home. That resulted in a lot of time yelling at each other while
she was in high school, and I would cry about
forever losing the closeness we had when she was
a little girl. I remember one year while she was
still in college, and I planned to stay in New
York for Thanksgiving because it followed an
education conference there the previous week.
I had always wanted to see the Macy's Thanksgiving Parade, and this was my opportunity. I
knew Elizabeth would come home for Thanksgiving, but I thought she would have Thanksgiving dinner with Kathryn and Ryan. Kathryn
called the week before I left to say that she and
Ryan and the little girls would be having Thanksgiving with Ryan's brother and she didn't know
if Elizabeth would want to go there. I hung up

the phone feeling guilty and then got mad because my life was not supposed to be like that. Dennis and I were supposed to be having all our children home to Dallas for Thanksgiving and the grown boys would be playing soccer in the front yard. Instead, I was living in Denton and planning Thanksgiving thousands of miles away from all my children.

When I walked back into the class I was teaching at the University of North Texas, one of my students asked me what was wrong because my eyes revealed sadness. I asked her to give me just a minute to come to terms with the fact that my life was different than what I thought it would be, she smiled and commented, "Well, you get two minutes, but just two. You are our role model for rising above adversity, so we have to know you are okay soon." Once again, a reminder to accept what was and to look at the message I was sending to others about living life.

Elizabeth remained in Austin for two and a half years after graduating from the University of Texas. She successfully created and managed a marketing position at a local sports bar before moving back to Dallas to become the event coordinator for a law firm. We made it through our tough times and now she is engaged to marry the young man she has dated for eight years. She asked me to give her away, and I can't think of anything that means more to me.

After putting himself through school for both his undergraduate and graduate degrees in finance, William is now taking classes to obtain his CPA to increase his career options. He and Nancy married four years ago and, with no children, travel frequently. He has a good life, and he is intentional about making time for what is important to him. For William, the loss was limited to his father's death because he didn't grow up with a stay-at-home mother whose life revolved around him. He joined our family at the age of eighteen and had a deep distrust of women caused by abandonment from his birth mother and abuse from the woman who had originally adopted him. After Dennis died, William realized he did have a steadfast love from me, and I was not going to abandon him. He has returned that love with support and pride for all my accomplishments.

In the end, just as I had to step back and allow my children to come to terms with their loss in each their own way, I also finally had to come to terms with the hard fact that grief recovery is a continuous journey. Even now, almost twenty years after I lost my beloved husband, any smell, sound, or word can take me back in an instant to the pain and sadness of 1995 and its aftermath. We live in a society that continually talks about closure, but what I've learned is that there really is no closure. Loss is like a hole in the heart, and although the hole becomes smaller, it never closes completely. I knew I could not spend the rest of my life wallowing in sadness, but losing my beloved Dennis to AIDS will always be part of who I am.

But I also realized something vitally important to my healing process. I found strength, continually, in finding ways to help others. As overwhelming as the initial loss was, the only way to keep going was to keep moving forward, and the only way to move forward was to not dwell on what was happening in my own grief but to look outward, find who or what needed my attention, and work from there. I could not have honored Dennis' memory and the life we had by doing anything differently.

But moving forward certainly didn't erase all events that continued to happen as a result of Dennis' death, and it certainly wasn't an easy journey. Five people grieving in different ways and at different levels of grief and at different times meant every word/every interaction could create an effect of bouncing from one person to another. As the surviving parent, sometimes I felt like I was a punching bag. I mean, who can blame a deceased parent for anything? When I thought the IRS might demand that I sell our house to pay the debt from unpaid taxes, Elizabeth, scared and unsure of the permanence of anything, was crying and yelling at me, and it hurt deeply. When Kathryn married and Samuel moved away, Elizabeth felt abandoned by her sister and her big brother, and nothing I said brought her any comfort.

It was another dimension to my own loss to witness the grieving of my children. As parents, we do everything we can to erase the hurt of our children. I so desperately wanted to make their hurt go away. For too long, I know my children felt like I was absent; although I felt like I was doing everything I could to make things better. They saw me as a completely different person from the mother they had known before their father died, and I expected them to see how my role had changed, so, of course, they would just flow with the changes. I wanted my children to understand my loss, as well as their own, but they were in too much pain to be able to understand anything outside of what they had lost. But because they thought the change had occurred in me and not in my role, I, too, believed that I was a different person than the one I had been the first forty-four years of my life.

My willingness and desire to help started early in my life. As a child with a mother who was often sick and a little sister I adored, I wanted to help by taking care of the people I loved. From my mother to my younger sister and older brother and then to Dennis' family and our children and my friends, I had spent my life taking care of the people I loved. When Dennis got sick, family and friends were immediately there taking care of us. I remember as a child, I was voted "prettiest eyes" and "friendliest" one summer at overnight camp. My mother told me to build on being friendly because that could make an ordinary life an extraordinary life. People took remarkable care of us while Dennis was sick and then after he died, and I know they helped me process my grief by their presence and by listening. A friend of mine gave me a book about women's friendships and in that book there was a chapter that had a letter from one experienced widow to a new widow. What the letter said, among other things, was to depend on friends for support, not family. Family was also grieving and could not be much help, but friends would get you through the rough days and nights. I depended on my friends, the friends I had when Dennis died and the friends I met in graduate school, and they never gave up on me.

Perhaps one of the most difficult parts for me was actually believing that Dennis was really gone. Eight years after his death, I was in my car driving to work after dropping Elizabeth off at school, and suddenly it hit me like a ton of bricks. This was the rest of my life. Dennis really wasn't coming back. I think that was when I began realizing I didn't have to keep fighting. I had been fighting to stay afloat for so many years, and I was tired. But somehow I finally knew we were not staying afloat, we were swimming strongly.

My role in life had changed, but I had not changed. Caring for my family, caring for my friends, caring for my students, I was the same person I had always been and that was a wonderful realization for me to have. It meant I had gotten through a horrific experience, but it had not destroyed me. I had always used the gifts given to me, and I would continue to use them. Shortly after Dennis died, I was sitting in church waiting for the worship service to begin. The words written for the personal prayer and meditation from the South Dalziel Parish Church resonated with me then, and I have carried them with me since that Sunday morning.

Since we cannot make the journey
backwards into innocence,
help us to go forward into wisdom.
Since we cannot begin again from the beginning,
help us to go on faithfully from here.
Since we cannot turn ourselves by our own will,
do Thou turn us towards Thee.

I had not been destroyed, but I was wiser and more intentional about living the life I had. Asking for strength, God has given me what I needed, and now I only need to be mindful of the opportunities for growth and use them. People have asked me how I could remember so much of the details about something that happened seventeen years ago. Losing my husband changed my life, and the details have not been forgotten.

I will never know why Dennis died the way he did, and I'll never know why my life ended up so differently from the life I thought I would have. As a young child, I wanted to be two things when I grew up—a trapeze artist and a mother. Running away to the circus never seemed to be an option, so I decided that "wife" would be an adventurous substitute. I wanted to marry and have children, to be involved in all that my family did. Looking back, I realized that I had been involved—until death do us part.

For the most part, I have stopped asking the questions for which there are no answers. What I do know is that I have built a life appreciating and caring for others and being appreciated and cared for in return. Instead of talking about my faith, I have tried to live my faith and that includes not only caring about people I know, but also caring about people I don't know, loving my neighbor as myself. I also know my mother was right. I had a chance to live an extraordinary life, and I took it. By faith, with family and with friends, *I have lived an extraordinary life.*

Acknowledgments

First, I'd like to thank my sister and brother-in-law, Judy and Marshall, for standing beside me from the beginning of this journey and never giving up on me. Every time I called Judy, she came with no hesitation. One day right before Dennis died, Marshall and I were alone, and I began crying. Marshall, instead of telling me to be strong, took me in his arms and let me cry. When I let go and he released me, my strength was replenished, and I knew I could keep breathing. My mother, Dottie Scott, and my brother, Arthur Scott, are both gone now, but who would I be if I did not mention them? Mother and Arthur were everything I needed them to be during this journey.

My heartfelt gratitude to my longtime friends Alice White and Becky Neeley, who stood with me before the diagnosis, stood with me during the journey of illness, and are standing with me today. They were my right and left hands while Dennis was sick, and since his death, they have celebrated every accomplishment with me.

On a hot summer day in July of 1995, Dave Neeley somehow knew that I was sinking. He quietly shepherded me with his strength and then whispered three words into my ear. Those three words became the anchor to my faith, the knowledge that as long as I kept going, God would not let me fail. Just keep breathing—thank you, Dave.

I could never have written this book without the belief and support and friendships of Carol Wickstrom and Veriena Braune. Carol and Veriena served as sounding boards for all the pieces in the telling of this story, and their compassion along with an unwavering belief in my resilience and my ability to write has provided the solid ground on which to stand when I felt unsure.

In 2003, I became part of The National Writing Project at a local site, The North Star of

Acknowledgments

Texas Writing Project. We teachers of writing work on learning more about the teaching of writing, as well as the writer in each of us. That summer, I wrote a six-page multi-genre paper about the death of my husband and finding a way to keep living. I had to make it multi-genre—obituary, lab slip, moving contract, etc.—because I did not have the words to really describe this deeply painful journey. Other teachers in this group have served as reflective editors for me as much of the writing of this book was accomplished during weekend writing retreats Leslie Patterson, Carol Revelle, Amanda Goss, and Polly Vaughan, thank you for believing, for supporting, and for suggesting.

Colleagues and others with whom I work have also been unending supporters. Thank you to Gail Frisby, Rachel Hawkins, Carolyn Matteson, Grace Anne McKay, Julie Tolle, and Barbara Vrana, for reading the unfinished manuscript, asking for clarifications so I knew where to fill holes, encouraging me to keep writing and finish the story. These women did more to support me than they realize.

For all the unnamed people who encouraged me to keep writing, I thank you. This is my story, but I have had the support of many people as I sought to tell it for others to read. Just like my life, I have had people helping all along the way.

A Message from the Author

I have read that we are the sum of our experiences. I believe that, at least for me. I cannot change what happened in my life, but I do have a choice in how I see the total result. Before I had firmly decided to try to publish this story, I used a piece of it to read aloud to teachers at the beginning of the school year. I talked about kindness and then I read a short selection from A. J. Palacio's *Wonder*, followed by a short selection from my own story. Both selections centered on kindness. I did not tell this group of teachers what I was reading.

At the break, one teacher approached me and asked if the second selection was my story. I asked her why she asked that question, and she answered, "Your voice is in that writing." I confirmed her suspicion, and I will never forget her response, "Dr. Curtis, you need to tell everyone here that that is your story. I am recently divorced and have been on food stamps. This is not a good time in my life. But I'm listening to you read about giving away your last twenty dollars, and I'm looking at you reading it, and my note to myself is Kel, you're not going to stay down. Look at her. Look at how far she's come. You'll do that, too, Kel. You will get out of this place."

That quick conversation cemented my decision. I cannot change what happened, but I can change what follows. I can open my eyes to all the miraculous moments and live them to the fullest. That is the message of my story. Life can be so difficult, so sad, at times, but keep your eyes open to the possibilities. I travelled by faith on this journey, never knowing what was going to happen, but trusting that someday I would be back in the light. I could never finish writing about every event, every choice, every decision, but I am always willing to share my story of living by faith.

Dr. Joan Scott Curtis,
Denton, Texas
January, 2013

www.ingramcontent.com/pod-product-compliance
Lightning Source LLC
Chambersburg PA
CBHW070758280326
41934CB00012B/2972